DH

Modifying
Vocal Behavior

UNDER THE ADVISORY EDITORSHIP

OF J. JEFFERY AUER

JOHN P. MONCUR

ISAAC P. BRACKETT

SOUTHERN ILLINOIS UNIVERSITY

Modifying Vocal Behavior

Harper & Row, Publishers

New York Evanston San Francisco London

Sponsoring Editor: Walter H. Lippincott, Jr.
Project Editor: Holly Detgen
Designer: Emily Harste
Production Supervisor: Stefania J. Taflinska

Modifying Vocal Behavior

Library of Congress Cataloging in Publication Data
Moncur, John P
    Modifying vocal behavior.

    1. Speech, Disorders of.   2. Speech therapy.
I. Brackett, Isaac P., joint author.   II. Title.
[DNLM: 1. Speech therapy.   2. Voice training.
WV500 M739m 1974]
RC427.M66   616.8′55   73–17669
ISBN 0–06–044567–X

To our wives,

Eva Beryl and Gwen

Contents

Preface

For many years speech clinicians in all types of employment situations have persistently asked for a text or manual of procedures and materials for the management of voice disorders. The request is not surprising since the study of voice disorders in training programs has primarily emphasized the anatomy, physiology, and scientific bases of normal voice production and the symptomatology, etiology, and diagnosis of voice disorders (including medical, surgical, and psychological considerations). Often, little attention has been directed to concerns of management and suggestions for treatment. Until quite recently, very few authors have addressed themselves directly to an in-depth consideration of approaches and procedures for different types of voice disorders.

The genesis of the present text was the desire to have in one place a compendium of procedures and materials to assist both the client and clinician in the modification of vocal behavior. In the early stages of preparing the text, a large corpus of procedures were sorted out under such general headings as relaxation, breathing, phonation, resonance, and prosody. Such an arrangement actually does little to provide the clinician with an approach to specific aspects of deviant vocal behavior. Indeed, it became clear that such an arrangement of material would influence the clinician to make a general or "wholistic" approach to management regardless of the distinctive nature of a voice problem; this would, in our opinion, be a serious mistake.

The authors agreed that discrete approaches should be made to specific voice problems, thereby encouraging a more molecular analysis. To do this, the clinician should be literally "led by the hand" in selecting procedures and materials for voice-problem management. In order to accomplish this task, it was apparent that a new, comprehensive framework based on a behavioral model was needed.

In *Modifying Vocal Behavior* we attempt to place management of voice disorders (disorders of the paracode) within a physiological and acoustical reference. The principles underlying such an approach embrace the concept that the physiological behaviors that directly generate the acoustics judged as a voice disorder should be the focus for modifying behaviors. All disorders of the paracode, regardless of the classification system, therefore, are disorders of function, because the behavior of the structures determine the acoustics.

The first five chapters of *Modifying Vocal Behavior* comprise the framework of reference for the management of voice disorders. Chapter 1 contains an overview of the physioacoustic parameters of voice production. Chapters 2 and 3 are devoted to the assessment of vocal behavior and the planning of the training program; Chapters 4 and 5 are concerned with modifying voice problems associated with laryngeal and cavity behaviors. Chapters 4 and 5 also refer the clinician to some of the more general procedures and approaches (e.g., relaxation, breathing, etc.) contained in the topical chapters, 6–10. Chapter 11 contains special procedures and approaches of a "wholistic" nature, such as the chewing method, the sustained voice approach, and the systematic desensitization in stimulus situations method of voice treatment, which are in common use today.

This text is conceived as a practical working guide or manual for the clinician who is trying to determine what to DO to help a client modify deviant vocal behavior; it is not conceived as a comprehensive academic presentation of voice disorders. For example, we have not attempted to include the usual information concerning incidence, pathology, diagnosis, surgery, psychology, extensive bibliographies, and so on, because standard texts and journal articles give adequate coverage to this type of information and are readily available. To do so would destroy the focus of the book.

We are keenly aware that physiological information, particularly as it is related to "the disorder," is not abundantly available and that there is much more information about such a condition or impairment as cleft palate than there is about its effect upon voice and speech. In writing this book it became abundantly clear to us that greater attention must be directed toward accumulating more complete information on the physioacoustics of vocal behavior. The present work, therefore, must be considered as only a beginning.

In summary, we have attempted to (a) assist the clinician and client in the clinical process; (b) provide a framework or classification system to permit more accurate descriptions and related physiologies of voice disorders; and (c) stimulate a further development of procedures, techniques, and materials for the management of voice disorders.

We are grateful to Mrs. Eva Beryl Moncur for her contribution to the book; namely, for her encouragement, writing creative sentences for drills, making suggestions concerning composition, and proofreading the manuscript.

We are indebted to Mrs. Gwen Brackett for her many efforts, which include a careful analysis of the first five chapters of the book, many suggestions, and hammering out typed manuscripts under the pressure of an early deadline.

Our appreciation is also extended to Dr. Gene J. Brutten for his suggestions concerning the systematic desensitization in stimulus situations procedures and the materials for managing vocal behavior found in Chapter 11.

Our thanks also go to our students, for requesting the information contained in *Modifying Vocal Behavior* and for their many stimulating questions—particularly those that probe toward new frontiers beyond our present knowledge.

J. P. M.
I. P. B.

Modifying
Vocal Behavior

1

The Physioacoustic Bases of the Code and Paracode

The various interpretations of the terms *voice* and *speech* reflect different aspects of verbal communication. *Voice* has served as a composite expression representing the total effect of speech, as a term limited to vibration of the vocal folds, and as a term referring to those acoustic parameters not directly related to the recognition of phonemes. *Speech* has also been used in the composite sense, as well as being restricted to the production and sequencing of phonemes (the "sounds" of words and phrases). The lack of specificity in the use of these two terms has resulted in some confusion in classifying disorders of verbal communication, which, in turn, has affected speech rehabilitation.

For the purposes of this text the word *speech* is used to mean the stream of composite physioacoustic events used by an individual for the purpose of verbal communication. The word *code* is used to mean those physioacoustic events within speech that make it possible for the listener (decoder) to identify the phoneme, word, or phrase. *Paracode* refers to all other speech phenomena that are not directly related to the identification of the word or phoneme, that is, frequency, intensity, quality, and duration in time. Speech, then, is the composite of two basic processes of verbal communication: (a) the *code*, or "what" is being said; and (b) the *paracode*, or "how" it is being said. The "what" and the "how" are both important to the decoder, for both contribute to meaningful speech. Generally speaking, all disorders of verbal communication affect the code or the paracode. Although the focus of this text is on the paracode, for the discussion of certain disorders, both the code and paracode will be considered.

Conceptualizing the code and paracode is important for those studying disorders of speech. However, it is essential to realize that these separate entities do not exist independently in the perception of the acoustics of speech. The code and paracode are not mutually independent, since the acoustic characteristics identifiable to the code coexist with, or are embedded in, those of the paracode. Assuming as a constant the ability to identify the phoneme, the variables of the paracode are those of quality, fundamental frequency, time or duration, and intensity. Consequently, a selected moment of a phoneme, such as a vowel, may contain (a) acoustics, or wave forms necessary to identify or decode the phoneme; (b) a fundamental frequency produced by varying modes of oscillation of the vocal folds; (c) acoustic variables described as quality (tonal, resonance); (d) an intensity; and (e) a time or duration of utterance. The code relates only to (a) above, while the paracode comprises all the other aspects listed. It is interesting to note that if all paracode attributes could be eliminated from speech, the code would cease to exist. Conversely, if all code factors were eliminated, the paracode would be meaningless sound. By sheer quantity of factors, the paracode possesses a greater potential for variation than the code and, to a large extent, accounts for individual differences between speakers. In "normal" speech, the production of the verbal code and paracode are within expected tolerances—that is, they do not deviate "too far" from an expected norm.

In discussing disorders or deviations from the norm of the code and paracode, judgments of the code differ from judgments of the paracode in that the former are more finite in terms of time and are restricted to given language units (i.e., the phoneme). Analysis of the paracode is much more general since it involves judgments over larger segments of time. If a judgment has been made of an event occurring during a period of time, then the same judgment may be made of a discrete moment. If a paracode judgment across time is that tonal quality is "breathy," then it follows that any voiced phoneme would have a breathy phonation; that is, voiced vowels, glides, nasals, plosives, fricatives, and affricates would display marked laryngeal turbulence. Perhaps those who are interested in the phoneme will begin talking about a hoarse "z," a fry "l," and a hypernasal "r." Phonemes can be described in their composite sense, in terms of both code and paracode variables.

Some of the traditional disorders of the paracode are not entirely manifest in short segments of time. Disorder classifications, such as "monopitch," unpredictable, sporadic phonation, inability to adapt vocal intensity to changes in situational demands, or tremulous phonation, are judgments not of the discrete moment but involve observations over longer periods of time. Single syllables are apt to be monopitch, or whispered, or soft, or loud. The disorder classification is based on a frequent recurrence of these characteristics over time.

DESCRIBING DISORDERS OF THE PARACODE

Judgments are made by the listener or decoder of the adequacy of the speaker's code or paracode. These judgments are basic to the clinical process. In describing what is being judged, it should be kept in mind that what is being listened to is a composite of acoustic events generated from a number of anatomic areas along the vocal tract, using a variety of physiological behaviors. Labeling has a tendency to create absolutes; once a label is assigned to one part of a composite, other parts are apt to be ignored. To say it another way, labels introduce a stasis into the dynamics of speech and speech disorders. It is also evident that many labels have become "dumping grounds" for a variety of physioacoustic events because of a lack of clarity in defining the terms for these events. Terms do not always mean the same thing to everybody, since they are symbols only and are subject to different interpretations.

Certainly, labels of paracode disorders reflect judgments by professional persons at moments in the clinical process. The difference in their labels are apt to be a reflection of their different concerns. The authors submit that, rather than depending on a single set of labels to record perceptions of disorders, descriptions of the physioacoustic events that constitute the disorder can be used to clarify the clinical process. Paracode disorders are value judgments by professional people and may be described in five different ways.

Descriptions of What Happens at Selected Moments of Speech

The terminology used describes changes noted in single phonemes, syllables, words, or phrases, such as omission, substitution, repetition, prolongation, and nasalization. This type of label is more frequently used in descriptions of disorders of the code, but it is also common in describing moments of stuttering behavior, as well as in certain aspects of voice quality.

Descriptions of Acoustic Characteristics

The terms used to describe the acoustics of a given sample of speech are of two basic types, physical and psychological. The physical terms describe the components of the signal that can be scientifically observed or measured —for example, frequency, intensity, and duration. The psychological terms reflect judgments of what the listener perceives—for example, breathy; psychological terms are subjective labels referring to a complex physical or psychological event.

Descriptions of Physiology

This type of terminology describes the motor behavior related to the perceived acoustic event—for example, the larynx is hypovalved, or there is insufficient excursion of the vocal folds, or the movements of the velopharyngeal sphincter are inadequate to close the velopharyngeal port.

Descriptions of the Condition of the Structures

This type of terminology refers to the impairment or change in the structures—for example, nodule, polyp, cleft palate, or paralysis. As in physiological descriptions, the terms result from visual inspection. The relationship between visual examination and acoustic product is, at this time, somewhat tenuous. For example, it is often assumed that hoarseness (an auditory impression) is a result of a pathology of the vocal folds. This may or may not be true, since hoarseness can also be a learned behavior.

Descriptions of Social and/or Psychological Relationships

Paracode disorders are also described from situational or interpersonal frames of reference. The effect "voice" has upon the listener is often noted —for example, a person's voice is said to be "too soft" or "too loud" or "grating." Generally, the problem is thought to be a function of relationships between individuals or the result of personal interaction. In hysterical aphonia, the inconsistencies of on-off phonation related to various situations or different subject matters are often attributed to difficulties in personal relationships; hence the term implies that the problem is psychological rather than pathological.

These five ways which form the bases of value judgments about paracode disorders may or may not be the problem. There are abundant examples in textbooks of disorders that are not disorders when they occur as people talk with one another. Speech problems become problems because someone is dissatisfied with his mode of speech production and desires change. All of the parameters of the paracode discussed in this text are potentially "normal" behaviors, given the appropriate circumstance or provided that no one makes them a problem. What is a problem under one set of circumstances may not be one under another set, because judgments are made both in situational contexts and from different points of view.

Actually, a speech disorder should only be described from the point of view of its effect on the verbal communication process. It would be inaccurate to call a vocal nodule or a congenital palatal insufficiency speech disorders, since these terms do not describe the effect of the "abnormality" on a speaker's verbal communication. When a disorder is described or labeled on the basis of many different judgments, the number of disorders may be multiplied. Once dissatisfaction has been expressed, complete understanding of the disorder often requires that it be examined from as many points of view as possible, using all available sources of information.

PHYSIOACOUSTICS OF THE CODE AND PARACODE

The preceding information assumes a listener is making judgments or classifying the acoustic attributes of a speaker's verbal communication. The acoustic output of the code and paracode is the *result* of relatively specific behaviors that modulate the airstream within the vocal tract. For the purposes of this text, *behavior* refers to the changes in vocal tract configurations that produce the wave forms relating to the acoustics of phonology. The code and paracode characteristics result from the behavior of anatomical structures. The same physiologies of airstream modulation account for the code characteristics in the sound envelope and the paracode characteristics. In the following pages, we review first the basic airstream modulations associated with speech and then those physiologies that are basic to wave form generation.

AIRSTREAM MODULATIONS

No human sound can be produced from the head and neck without (a) a reservoir of air, such as that supplied at the lungs after inhalation; and (b) the ability to create a flow of air of sufficient amount. Given these two basic requirements, the attributes of the code and paracode result from three basic airstream modulations: (a) the acoustics associated with pressure release, (b) the acoustics of air turbulence (frication), and (c) the acoustics associated with vibrating structures.

The Acoustics of Pressure Release

The acoustics associated with pressure release are the product of a complete closure of the vocal tract at some point; this closure permits a build-up of air pressure. When the closure is released, the sudden escape of positive air pressure, with its turbulence, accounts for the acoustic event often described as a "plosive." Complete closure of the vocal tract can be achieved at the vocal folds (laryngeal valving), by the tongue against the posterior pharyngeal wall, by the tongue anywhere along the roof of the mouth, and by the lips pressed together or against the teeth. When the closure is within the oral cavity, the build-up of pressure also requires a closure of the velopharyngeal sphincter. Effecting closures at different anatomical areas change the vocal tract characteristics into which the pressure is released. Therefore, assuming the same amount of pressure release, the difference between a [k] and a [t] is partly a difference in cavity dimensions. Also, changing the dimension of the cavities for any vowel that follows the pressure release will change the characteristics of the [k] or [t]. That is, a [k] released into a cavity shaped for an [i] is acoustically different from a [k] released into a cavity shaped for an [æ], since the pressure release is into two different vocal tract configurations.

The code and paracode characteristics relating to pressure release are associated with voiceless plosives ([p], [t], [k], [ʔ]). When pressure release is used to initiate the phonation of voiced phonemes, the terms glottal shock, coup de glotte, or hard attack are used. The hard attack is characteristic of individuals speaking with hyperlaryngeal valving (strident-harsh tonal quality).

The Acoustics of Air Turbulence

Air turbulence results from narrowing the vocal tract at some point, and, if airflow is sufficient, the resistance supplied by the constriction causes the airstream to whirl or eddy. The amount of constriction, its shape, and the quantity of the airflow determine the amount of turbulence. The shape and size of the cavity spaces into which the turbulence escapes vary the acoustics, since air turbulence, like pressure release, excites resonators. If the constricture of the tract is within the oral cavity, the airflow route requires the closure of the velopharyngeal sphincter to be greater than the degree of constriction of any of the other orifices along the vocal tract. Otherwise, major air direction would be altered since airflow follows the route of least resistance.

The code and paracode characteristics associated with air turbulence are many and varied. Turbulence is one of the more common acoustics in verbal communication. Voiceless fricatives, [f], [θ], [s], [ʃ], are identified as code characteristics of turbulence. When combined with pressure release, turbulence accounts for the affricates, [ts], [ks], [ps], [tʃ]. The [h] as a voiceless vowel[1] is fascinating to study, for the turbulence associated with its production is directly related to the shape of the cavity for the phonated vowel that follows. If, for example, the tongue constricts the oral cavity, as in the high vowels [i] or [u], the turbulence is within the oral cavity, whereas for a low vowel [ɑ] the turbulence is generated at the level of the glottis. Variations in turbulence and pressure release account for all speech characteristics of whisper. Turbulence as an airstream modulation is responsible for the paracode attributes of quality, such as breathiness, and is certainly part of the composite acoustics of hoarseness or other dysphonias. When speech seems to be excessively turbulent (excessive airflow), short phrases often result. The voice may be described as having insufficient loudness, and the vocal personality described as one of shyness or timidity. To some, excessive turbulence is an air "wastage" problem, and behavioral change is concentrated on better control during exhalation.

The Acoustics of Vibrating Structures

The ability of structures, such as the vocal folds, to vibrate completes this discussion of the acoustic requirements of verbal communication. When structures comprised chiefly of soft tissues are moved into or across the stream of air, the resistance causes pressure increase (providing the pressure flow is great enough), which pushes the structures apart. The negative pressure resulting from the sudden release of airflow will then bring the structures toward each other (Bernoulli effect), creating cycles of vibration. This oscillation of the structures generates the sound waves commonly referred to as laryngeal phonation.

---

[1] The [h] has been traditionally classified as a glottal fricative; however, the very nature of [h] decrees that it is more justifiably classified as a voiceless vowel.

Phonation involves a number of characteristics of the sound composite of speech. The number of oscillations in a given period of time provides a fundamental frequency, which is often described in terms of pitch. Variations in tension, mass, and length of the vocal folds and in subglottic air pressure give the potential for a range of fundamental frequencies. In addition, various modes of oscillation, such as fry and falsetto, extend the range potential higher or lower than the range of "normal" oscillation. Obviously, the vibrating structures will increase the energy characteristics of phonated speech versus whispered speech, for example, and the regularity or irregularity of their vibrating patterns will determine the quality described as tonal (harmonic) or noise (inharmonic).

The vibrating structures of the vocal folds are within connected cavity spaces and therefore excite the air mass in cavities and give rise to the physical phenomenon of resonance. Resonance changes caused by modifying the dimensions, openings, and couplings of cavities account for both the code characteristics of vowels and consonants and for quality differences in voices as well. Sound waves generated by the vibration of the vocal folds and amplified in the resonating cavities permit the doubling of plosives, fricatives, and affricates. Phonation, although an independent variable in the sound composite of speech, plays a dominant role in the production of the code and paracode. Where an examination is made of the acoustics of the paracode, the importance of vibrating structures is evident, for they are ultimately related to quality, loudness or energy, frequency or pitch, and rate of duration. It is no wonder phonation and voice are synonymous for many professional persons. It must also be kept in mind that the contributions of vocal fold vibration are germane to the code as well as the paracode.

MAJOR PHYSIOLOGIES OF THE PARACODE

The variables of the paracode are directly attributable to four major physiological continua: (a) the continuum of laryngeal valving; (b) the behaviors of the vibrator, that is, the continuum of fundamental frequencies and amplitudes produced by various modes of vocal fold oscillation; (c) the continuum of resonating cavity dimensions, openings, and textures; and (d) the continuum of nasal couplings. These same continua could also be discussed with reference to the code, but that is not within the scope of this text. The relation of these major physiological continua to the disorders of voice will be discussed in Chapters 4 and 5. They are described below in an effort to form a basis for clinical judgments.

Laryngeal Valving

The various positions of the vocal folds between complete abduction and complete adduction provide a variety of tonal or atonal qualities, described as whisper, breathy, optimal, and strident (harsh). The schematic diagram in Figure 1.1 illustrates this continuum. The degree of valving referred to as "optimal" represents the majority of phonations for verbal communication. Normal phonation may deviate in either direction depending on the criteria of normalcy. The term optimal is used to identify valving that permits the most efficient vibration of the vocal folds.

The *hypovalved larynx* is distinguished by its acoustics of turbulence caused by the narrowing of the passage and the low resistance to airflow. Of course, when the vocal folds are in the completely abducted position, the laryngeal valve is contributing nothing to airstream modulation; hence, any sound generated would be localized to other areas along the vocal tract, as in buccal speech (oral compression of air). The laryngeal air turbulence occurs when either the true vocal folds or the ventricular folds are partially valved, as in the whisper, or when the vocal folds are partially valved and vibrating, as in hypovalvular phonation.

The *optimally valved larynx* is evidenced by its "clear" phonation produced by free, unhampered, periodic vibration of the vocal folds. A *hypervalved larynx* is noted for its penetrating phonation and increased struggle behavior to initiate phonation—hence the labels "harsh," "metallic," or "pinched throat."

The clinical judgments relating to laryngeal valving and its tonal or atonal qualities are at times complicated by the presence of a laryngeal pathology.

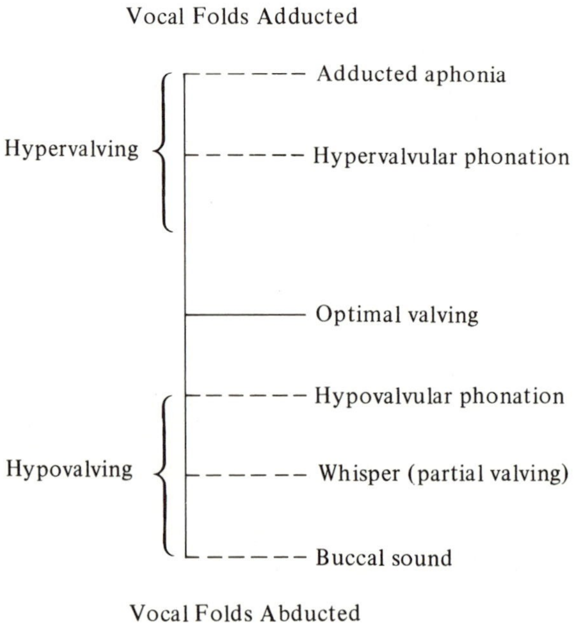

Figure 1.1
Continuum of laryngeal valving.

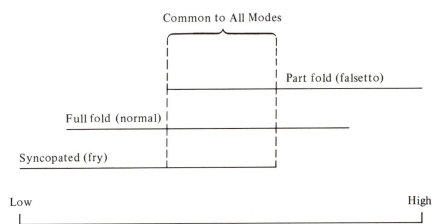

Figure 1.2
The modes of vocal-fold oscillation.

This is especially true when the pathological condition prevents the vocal folds from approximating adequately and the speaker hypervalves the vocal folds in an effort to compensate. The result is turbulence *and* stridency, both of which are aspects of laryngeal noise.

Laryngeal Oscillation

There are at least three modes, or registers,[2] of vocal fold oscillation: full fold (normal); part fold, or falsetto; and syncopated, or fry. Each of these modes generates a range of fundamental frequencies within the spectrum of fundamental frequencies common to the three modes. Figure 1.2 illustrates the range of fundamental frequencies for each mode of oscillation. Note that there is a range of frequencies common to all three modes—that is, the ranges of fry, full fold, and falsetto overlap. Within each mode of oscillation and its potential range, speakers generally have a modal frequency (i.e., a frequency that is more commonly used than others), with fluctuation around the modal frequency relating to the range use.

Judgments of laryngeal oscillation relate to (a) the mode of oscillation and its appropriateness, (b) the position of the modal frequency within range use and the range potential, and (c) whether use of the frequency range is appropriate to the communication intent. One important aspect of oscillation is amplitude of vocal fold vibration, which determines, in part,

---

[2] The term register has been used in different contexts, as a resonance or quality phenomenon of the chest or head or as different modes of oscillation of the vocal folds. It is in the latter context that the authors employ this term throughout the text.

the intensity of the signal. Amplitude is the product of the degree of laryngeal valving, the intrinsic tension of the vocal folds, the mode of oscillation, and the amount of subglottal breath pressure or airflow. Assuming a constant airflow from the lungs, the more optimal the valving, the greater the amplitude of vibration. Extremes of hypovalving and hypervalving seriously affect the amplitude of the vibration. In addition, the amplitude potential is reduced with part fold (falsetto) or syncopated (fry) oscillation.

Laryngeal Noise

The generation of laryngeal noise, commonly referred to as "husky," "hoarse," or "rough" phonation, is the result of three basic physiologies: (a) laryngeal hypovalving, which results in air turbulence; (b) laryngeal hypervalving, which produces a harsh-strident phonation; and (c) irregular vibration of the vocal folds or surrounding structures, which results in aperiodic phonation. No two composites of laryngeal noise in individuals are exactly alike because different proportions of these physiological conditions are used. Often associated with laryngeal noise are sudden changes in the mode of oscillation, which create marked shifts in fundamental frequency (pitch breaks), from falsetto to normal or from fry to normal or falsetto. Occasionally, two fundamental frequencies may be produced simultaneously (diplophonia); this may be associated with other aspects of laryngeal noise.

DIMENSIONS, OPENINGS, AND TEXTURES OF RESONATING SPACES

The wave forms generated by laryngeal behaviors are released into supraglottal resonating spaces. The code characteristics unique to a specific phoneme are largely the product of cavity variables, especially those of the oral cavity. But aside from wave forms directly related to the identification of a phoneme, the resonating spaces contribute a dimension of resonant quality. Differences in resonant quality among individuals are the product of (a) differences in cavity dimensions, (b) differences in openings into and out of the cavity spaces, (c) differences in texture (hardness or softness of walls), and (d) whether the nasal air route is coupled or uncoupled to the pharyngo-oral system.

Cavity Dimensions

The size, length, or shape of the cavity determines certain aspects of resonance. Generally speaking, the larger the cavity, the greater the amplification of lower formant resonance frequencies. Conversely, the smaller the cavity, the greater the amplification of higher formant characteristics. The pharyngo-oral dimensions can be changed by (a) high or low position of the larynx; (b) contraction or expansion of the pharyngeal cavity; (c) front or back position of the tongue and jaw in the oral cavity; and (d) position of the soft palate or velum. Physiological changes that give maximum size or length to cavity space produce resonance characteristics commonly labeled "muffled," "retracted," or "throaty," while changes that reduce cavity size or length result in quality attributes referred to as "oral," "thin," or "immature." Immature quality is often confused with "high pitch" or "high" fundamental frequency, and behavioral change is inappropriately directed toward lowering pitch rather than increasing the size of the resonator or decreasing the size of openings.

Cavity Openings

The openings into and out of cavities can be varied by (a) the position of the jaw and lips, (b) the forward or backward posturing of the tongue in the oral cavity, (c) the height of the tongue in the oral cavity in its posturing for the vowel, and (d) the position of the velum in readiness for speech. Generally, smaller openings into or out of a resonator amplify the lower formant characteristics, and larger openings amplify the higher formant characteristics. Therefore, the qualities "muffled," "retracted," or "throaty" result not only from large cavities but also from smaller openings from the pharynx into the oral cavity or at the mandible or lips. Conversely, those qualities referred to as "oral," "thin," or "immature" result from smaller cavities and larger openings.

Texture of Walls

The surface tension, that is, hardness or softness, of the walls of a resonator undoubtedly contributes to the frequency response of cavities. The more rigid the walls, the greater the amplification of higher resonance formants; the softer the walls, the greater the emphasis of the lower resonance formants. In the human being, the ability to voluntarily change the characteristics of the walls of resonators is limited. It should be noted, however, that contraction and relaxation of antagonistic muscle groups "tighten" or "soften" the surface status of resonators. In those areas of the vocal tract where muscle fibers make up a part of the wall structure, as in the pharynx and the oral cavity, these changes in surface tension do contribute to the quality characteristics of the paracode. The hypervalving of the larynx, especially of the ventricular folds, not only affects the size of the laryngopharynx but also the surface tension of the walls. Other factors, like swelling or edema related to conditions of inflammation or infection, also change the surface and size characteristics.

COUPLING AND UNCOUPLING THE NASAL PASSAGE

The discussion of the resonance characteristics of the pharyngo-oral air route assumes that the nasal air passage is closed by the velopharyngeal sphincter (uncoupled). The coupling of the nasal resonators to the pharyngo-oral resonating system adds other resonance characteristics to the sound envelope. The resonance of the nasal air spaces are referred to as nasal resonance if accompanied by laryngeal phonation (vocal fold vibration) and as nasal air turbulence if the nasal spaces are excited by extremes of airflow.

To produce the code characteristics of [m], [n], and [ŋ], the nasal air passages must be coupled to the pharyngo-oral system so that, with vocal fold vibration, nasal resonance will result. The three nasal sounds are then differentiated by varying amounts of cul-de-sac oral resonance. Without vocal fold vibration, air turbulence is largely generated within the narrow nasal passages (producing nasal emission or a voiceless nasal fricative). Without other cues such as vision, it is difficult to recognize acoustic differences between the three whispered nasal sounds. If the nasal air route cannot be coupled to the pharyngo-oral system because of a blockage, the [m], [n], and [ŋ] become similar to the voiced plosives [b], [d], and [g]. When changes such as these occur in the nasal sounds, the terms negative nasality, denasality, hyponasality, and rhinolalia clausa posterior are used to describe the effect.

There are instances when the negative effect of blocked nasal passages and the positive effect of hypernasality on vowels exist at different moments in the flow of speech. For example, a blockage near the front of the nasal passage accompanied by a mild insufficiency of the velopharyngeal sphincter results in a voiced plosive effect on the nasal phonemes (code change) and a hypernasal effect from the cul-de-sac nasal resonance on vowels and glides (paracode). The combination of positive and negative aspects of nasal coupling is referred to as rhinolalia clausa anterior, or *mixta*.

All other code characteristics of speech—the vowels, glides, plosives, fricatives, and affricates—do not require a coupling of the nasal air passage for the listener to identify the phoneme. When degrees of coupling occur during moments of non-nasal code production, the effect is described as positive nasality, hypernasal resonance, or rhinolalia aperta. When the nasal air route is coupled on the vowels and glides, the perceived nasal resonance is an attribute of the paracode; but when nasal coupling is present during the production of plosives, fricatives, and affricates, it is classified as a code disorder because the identification of the phoneme is adversely affected. The presence of hypernasality on the vowels and glides usually does not interfere with phoneme recognition, unless it is extreme, but hypernasality does interfere with the recognition of plosives, fricatives, and affricates.

Individuals who possess hypernasality can be divided into three groups: (a) those whose nasal resonance is apparent on vowels adjacent to the nasal continuant only (assimilated nasality); (b) those whose nasal resonance is apparent on glides and vowels, especially high vowels, regardless of the presence of a nasal phoneme, but whose other code characteristics are produced satisfactorily; and (c) those whose nasal resonance and emission affect the code characteristics of the plosives, fricatives, and affricates, with or without hypernasality on vowels and glides.

As a model, the expected effect of nasal coupling on plosives, fricatives, and affricates might be summarized in the following manner: (a) All voiced plosives, fricatives, and affricates appear similar to positionally related nasal continuants. (b) All voiceless plosives, fricatives, and affricates become voiceless nasal fricatives (nasal emission). Naturally, various degrees of incompetency of the velopharyngeal sphincter and learned compensatory behaviors will alter this model; therefore, complete speech assessment is indicated.

SUMMARY

The purpose of this chapter is to present a general overview of the physioacoustic parameters of the paracode and of the code when indicated. This overview should provide a reference for subsequent chapters, which consider in detail those variations of verbal communication judged to be disorders of the paracode.

2

Assessing
Vocal Behaviors

The purpose of vocal assessment is to ascertain whether vocal behaviors can be modified. Complete assessment of the client involves (a) formal procedures to provide insights into the cause and extent of the disorder (i.e., medical diagnoses, tests, case history, relevant reports); (b) vocal assessment procedures that explore the parameters of voice to determine the physioacoustic manifestations of the problem; and (c) techniques to ascertain whether behavioral change is possible. Each of these is basic to the process of determining and planning a course of behavior change.

The time required to obtain the necessary information varies considerably because of the wide range of differences in voice problems. In some instances, as with clients who have had a laryngectomy, assessment and treatment are apt to be one and the same. Outside of obtaining basic information for the record, the clinician should start at once trying to teach esophageal phonation and buccal speech. Conversely, judgments cannot be made in certain cases until certain information is accumulated (x-rays, reports, etc.) and, therefore, vocal assessment may be delayed. It is possible that with some clients (e.g., a cleft palate child) the documentation of the extent of the disorder is prolonged over a number of years before final disposition can be completed. In most instances, the assessment of disorders of the paracode can be completed in relatively short periods of time, and a course of action implemented.

Since the chief purpose of vocal assessment is to decide whether behavior of the paracode can be modified, all materials and procedures used should be directed toward assisting the clinician to render an accurate professional judgment. For this reason, the present chapter has been organized in the following temporal sequence: (a) initial contact, (b) analysis of the complaint or request, (c) assessment of vocal behavior, (d) experimental programs to estimate prognosis, and (e) disposition.

NATURE OF THE INITIAL CONTACT

Clients come to the clinician's attention in a variety of ways, which can structure, in part, the professional intervention. Should the clinician be a staff member of an organization such as a hospital, client contacts are handled as a routine procedure. But when the clinician is an independent professional, the manner of the initial contact will vary considerably. Speech clinicians should be aware of the different roles they play in the contact. Initial contacts may be grouped under these general headings: (a) located by the clinician, (b) professional referral, (c) referred or brought by an interested person, and (d) self-referral.

Located by Clinician

Perhaps the most common "case finding" is accomplished by screening. The public health concept is to locate the health care problems within society, ascertain the extent of the problems, and establish procedures (i.e., referral) that will eradicate or prevent the problems from recurring. Primarily for this reason, screening for speech, vision, hearing, and other problems is conducted within school systems on a regular basis. The speech clinician identifies possible clients by this screening process. It needs to be understood that the standards used to make judgments of possible disorders during screening are those of the clinician. Not all problems identified in this manner will be substantive ones, since criteria of defective speech are not always the same. The clinician should recognize that apparent speech problems that are revealed in screening should be discussed with the parents of the children and perhaps the classroom teacher to see if there is a concern and a desire for professional assistance. No child should be scheduled in a formal training program without the full understanding and approval of the child's parents or guardian.

Professional Referral

Professional referral is an important way for clients to come to the attention of the speech clinician. In professional referral, one professional person is seeking the help of another—for example, a teacher, doctor, lawyer, or psychologist requests professional intervention from a speech clinician. These requests are generally of two types: (a) to render a professional opinion as a service to the professional person making the referral, and (b) to begin professional treatment. In the first instance, the opinion is usually rendered in a report or orally in a consultation, and once the report is given, client contact is terminated. In the second instance, however, both the referring person and the client expect professional services to be rendered by the speech clinician for an appropriate period of time and to a specific end. There are instances, for example, when voice behavior change is performed as a part of and in conjunction with medical treatment, and a professional team situation prevails. The speech clinician needs to understand the various possible professional relationships and to perform accordingly.

Referred or Brought by an Interested Person

Very often, a person close to a client will recommend that he be seen for professional advice concerning his problem and may be responsible for taking him to the clinic. The most frequent example of this type of referral is within family groups—for example, parents bring their child to the speech clinician because of their concern. It is important for the speech clinician to respond quickly to these informal referrals, for the people requesting help are usually concerned and feel frustrated if delay is prolonged.

Self-referrals

Self-referred persons are usually highly motivated because (a) they recognize the need for professional services and (b) they have, by whatever means, gone to the source they think can best help them. In many ways, this is complimentary and supportive to the remedial program, but there may be times when the needs of the client cannot be fully met, and the clinician then acts as a referral agent to the appropriate professional person.

Each type of initial contact carries unique obligations to the speech clinician. The ethics of the profession establish the guidelines for appropriate responses to individuals requesting services. Subsequent to the initial contact, the speech clinician should schedule the time necessary to conduct an adequate assessment of the problem.

ANALYSIS OF THE COMPLAINT OR REQUEST

Complaints about voice or speech production range from vague expressions of dissatisfaction to specific requests for assistance to achieve desired goals—from "There is something wrong with the way he talks" to "My child has a hoarse voice and needs therapy." In the first instance, the speech clinician must determine the exact nature of the complaint. This usually means preliminary discussions with the interested persons to discover what provokes the comment. In the second instance, formal assessment procedures can be initiated.

Whenever possible, the speech clinician should respond to the expressed needs of the client as tempered by professional judgments. It is not uncommon for the clinician to be aware of possible problems of speaking (code or paracode) that are not complained about by the client or, if the client is a child, by members of his family. These should be discussed to determine the interest, desire, or motivation to pursue the matter further. In this same vein, the problem may not appear as critical to the clinician as it does to the client, and counseling is the indicated response to the request.

There will also be occasions when professional judgment decrees that the client be seen for another type of service (e.g., medical, psychiatric, etc.), which may override the needs expressed by the individual. This is especially true when the speech clinician suspects a condition like cancer or papillomas and urges medical evaluation.

Being attentive to the nature of the complaint and resolving differences of opinion that may exist enable the speech clinician to begin accumulating the information needed to form the bases of professional judgments. Because of differences in initial contacts, some clients have already been thoroughly "diagnosed," and extensive information is available to the clinician. With other clients, the burden of information gathering is left entirely to the clinician. Prior to the assessment of vocal behavior, therefore, the clinician may have to assemble or develop pertinent data, such as previous examinations by professional persons, the results of tests administered, records of previous therapy, and case history information directly related to the disorder.

The professional literature contains an abundance of case history forms, examination procedures, and other suggestions for gathering this type of information that will not be duplicated here. Clinicians vary from those with an almost compulsive need to have a complete file of information about the client to those who merely make a hurried judgment about the needs of the client and begin a program of training with little understanding of the behaviors that need to be changed. The authors urge that information be specific as to what is required to render an accurate opinion. The nature of the disorder, the information gleaned from the initial contact, and the availability of other sources of professional information will determine the extent of time devoted to information gathering.

Based upon knowledge about the individual with the voice disorder, including a general impression of the problem from listening to the client, the clinician ascertains the procedures and materials needed for the assessment of vocal behaviors. The procedures and materials should be specifically selected to suit the problem. The clinician should not ask the client to perform tasks that do not contribute directly to the information needed for decision-making, simply because they are part of a routine diagnostic procedure. Ordinarily, the procedures and materials are selected or developed by the clinician because of their worth to the assessment of the particular disorder.

ASSESSMENT OF VOCAL BEHAVIORS

The clinician, with information assembled from the initial contact, proceeds with an analysis of vocal behaviors associated with paracode disorders. Even if other professional persons have described or labeled the client's disorder, it is wise to conduct one's own analysis. Although the focus of the analysis is usually a particular behavior, it is desirable that the clinician examine all parameters of the paracode in the process of assessment. Assume, for example, that because of perceived hypernasality, the principal behavior under question is the adequacy of the velopharyngeal sphincter. At times, however, other physioacoustic events, such as laryngeal hyper-valving, may accentuate the perception of hypernasality. Therefore, assessing all parameters of the paracode provides an insight into other attributes of the vocal composite and assists in identifying other behaviors that also may need to be modified. Disorders are rarely the result of a single physiological event.

The clinician should evaluate the parameters of the paracode in a systematic, routine manner. Depending on the disorder, certain aspects of the routine may be passed over quickly, while others receive more time for analysis; but, still, all physioacoustic parameters should be surveyed. The assessment program should include: (a) breathing for speech and its adequacy to provide a reservoir and airflow potential; (b) laryngeal valving; (c) behavior of the vibrator (i.e., mode of oscillation, fundamental frequency, and amplitude); (d) the dimensions, openings, and couplings of resonators; and (e) prosody characteristics, such as use of pitch changes, quality, rate, and loudness.

Adequacy of Breath for Speech

Observation should be directed to the quantity of air intake prior to speech, the movements of exhalation (thoracic, abdominal, etc.) and their duration, any difficulty in airflow direction, and opinions on the adequacy of breathing for speech.

PROCEDURES

1. Observe the quantity of air intake and the movements of exhalation. Use the procedures for evaluating central control on pp. 128–132.
2. Explore the depth and control of breathing, pp. 132–134.
3. For the client who hypovalves his larynx, observe breath supply and wastage of air, pp. 134–135.
4. Evaluate the adequacy of breathing for pauses and phrases, including different phrase lengths, pp. 135–140.
5. Evaluate the adequacy of breath supply and control for loudness, pp. 140–144.

Laryngeal Valving

The status of vocal fold posturing during speech should be evaluated, including the ability to initiate phonation, the appropriateness of on-off phonation to phoneme production, and a general description of the tonal or atonal quality.

PROCEDURES

1. Evaluate voice production while the client reads sentences with contrasting voiced and voiceless phonemes.
2. Evaluate voice production while the client performs sentences of different length; pay particular attention to the ends of sentences.
3. Have the client read several sentences with a number of words beginning with vowels (e.g., *I ate an apple*) in order to evaluate vocal attack, pp. 149–150.
4. Have the client laugh, clear his throat, and cough in order to make judgments of his ability to vary the status of valving.
5. Explore the ability of the client to use contrast behaviors in valving, that is, hypervalve the hypovalved larynx and hypovalve the hypervalved larynx, p. 150.
6. Refer to Chapters 4 and 9 for additional information and materials.

Behaviors of the Vibrator

Assessment of the behaviors of the vibrator includes (a) the mode or modes of oscillation, (b) precipitous and unexpected changes in mode of oscillation, (c) modal fundamental frequency, (d) the relative position of the modal frequency within the use range and the range potential, (e) an estimate of tonal quality, and (f) the adequacy of the amplitude of the vibrator.

PROCEDURES

1. Have the client read a paragraph of sufficient length in order to make appropriate judgments concerning pitch and pitch changes.
2. Use a piano or pitch pipe to ascertain extent of range.
3. If modal pitch seems too high or too low, determine optimum pitch, pp. 65–69.
4. Ask the client to vary vocal loudness while sustaining a vowel.
5. Observe voice quality while the client hums a tone. Experiment with different pitch levels.
6. Refer to Chapter 1 for information on the physiology of the vibrator and to Chapters 6 and 9 for additional information and material.

Dimensions and Openings

Certain characteristic uses of resonators can be observed: (a) the position of the thyroid cartilage during phonation, (b) the extent of the movement of the mandible during vowel production, and (c) the general posturing of the tongue forward or back in the mouth. Visual information should be related to the perceived acoustics, since changes in cavity dimensions and openings relate to the oral-pharyngeal resonant qualities, oral-thin-immature or guttural-muffled-retracted-throaty.

PROCEDURES

1. Listen to the quality of the vowels and glides while the client is reading.
2. Judge the predominance of high or low resonance during phonation.
3. Listen to fricatives and affricates, since their acoustic characteristics differ in relation to tongue posturing in the oral cavity (i.e., high resonance produces "sharp s's" while low resonance produces "dull s's").
4. Refer to Chapters 5 and 10 for additional information and materials.

Couplings

In assessing the nature of positive nasal coupling, attention should be directed to the quality of the vowels and glides and the production of the plosives, fricatives, and affricates.

PROCEDURES

1. Use selected words and carefully designed sentences that permit an evaluation of the effect of vowel height, p. 181.
2. Evaluate voice quality while the client performs high and low vowels initiated by different consonants.
3. Evaluate voice quality while the client performs sentences composed of different sequences of phonemes (e.g., all low vowels and glides, all high vowels with fricatives and affricates).
4. Judge the ability of the client to manage various combinations in sequential speech using various types of clusters to establish the extent of the velopharyngeal incompetence and its effect on speech.
5. Refer to Chapters 5 and 10 for additional information and materials.

Negative nasal coupling (denasal as well as *mixta*) can best be assessed during conversation or by asking the client to read short paragraphs that contain a repetition of the nasal phonemes.

General Prosody Characteristics

In all vocal assessment situations, it is desirable to observe the function of other vocal parameters, such as pitch variations, rate, loudness, and quality, over an extended period of time. These should be judged with respect to the appropriateness to the subject matter, the situation, and the aspirations or needs of the client. It is important to know the vocal objectives of clients, since use of voice to achieve certain ends must always be kept in mind. The clinician should make note of sudden inappropriate changes in prosody.

PROCEDURES

1. Make a tape recording of the client reading a prose passage.
2. Study the use of various pitch functions (range, pitch contours, etc.) to determine their appropriateness. Use the materials in Chapter 6 to assist with the evaluation.

3. Assess rate in terms of duration of phonemes, syllables, words, phrases, sentences, and overall rate, pp. 90–96.
4. Assess the use of force for stress, overall intensity level, variety, and projection, pp. 97–102. Present a variety of speaking situations (e.g., large and small rooms) and evaluate the appropriateness of the client's use of general intensity level in each.
5. Make an evaluation of the combined use of all of the factors of prosody to express meaning and emotion.

EXPERIMENTAL PROGRAMS

At some time, the clinician should attempt to modify the client's vocal behavior by means of an experimental program to estimate the potential for improvement. In this way, the clinician determines whether professional speech intervention can be successful. It also permits the clinician to describe the desired approach to modification by delineating the behavior that can be achieved and strengthened. Experimental programs may also be used to probe further into the nature of the problem, particularly where the initial assessment was not conclusive.

Based on the procedures for assessment of vocal behaviors just described, the specific behaviors that are basic to the disorder should be identified. The purpose of experimental procedures is to see if the client can initiate contrasting behaviors to those associated with the disorder. For example, if the larynx is hypervalved (strident), can the client hypovalve the larynx to produce a breathy phonation? If the client can change toward the contrasting behavior, prognosis is favorable and scheduling of formal speech sessions would appear warranted. However, if no contrasting behavior can be initiated, prognosis is unfavorable and continued training is contra-indicated. The clinician may elect to continue the experimental procedures for a longer period of time to see if contrasting behaviors can be initiated. This approach should be applied to all behavior associated with the disorder. If the clinician cannot initiate a change of behavior, it is apparent that (a) further diagnosis is indicated, and referral should be made to the appropriate professional person (medical, etc.); or (b) solving the problem may not be within the competency of the clinician, and further professional responsibility should be terminated either by counseling or by referral to a professional person with different or greater skills.

DISPOSITION

The assessment should conclude with a documentation of the procedures used and the judgments made. This is usually a short report with the pertinent information, including dates of contacts and other routine information. It is wise to write a description of the assessment, however brief, for the record, since reference to the contact will undoubtedly be needed in the future.

The disposition of the case after assessment entails implementing the results of the professional opinion in response to the type of service requested. Various possible dispositions are described in the following list.

1. Write a report documenting in detail the bases of the professional opinion and recommendations; make the report available to the authorized professional person approved by the client. This action may terminate any further professional relationship with the client.
2. Refer the client to another professional for further diagnosis to determine the extent of the disorder. This is usually the option if the assessment has been inconclusive, and the need for further information is indicated. Actually, the assessment is incomplete, and the case is held pending further information. Hopefully, the delay is only for a short period.
3. Refer the client to another professional colleague for treatment, or determine if the client would be better served if treatment were shared with another professional. Shifting or sharing the responsibility for training should be accomplished without too much delay and to the complete satisfaction of the client.
4. Schedule the client for an experimental program of assessment. If the inappropriate vocal behavior of the client can be changed, as determined by an experimental program of training, a formal remedial program can be instituted. Termination of treatment shall be at the discretion of the clinician and/or his client, when it is determined that further work would not be beneficial to the client.
5. Terminal counseling may need to be considered when it is abundantly clear that voice training would not be beneficial to the client. At times, it is important that the client realize that adjustment to the disorder is more important than futile efforts to eradicate it. Of course, the client may wish to seek other professional assistance, but should this not be desired, the only alternative may be in counseling the client in ways to manage everyday situations to his satisfaction in spite of the vocal disorder. Learning to live with a disability is a challenge, and a speech clinician can be extremely helpful in the adjustment process.

SUMMARY

The purpose of this chapter is to establish general procedures for assessing vocal behaviors. Clinicians are encouraged to take the necessary time to evaluate clients before commiting themselves to continuing professional relationships to modify vocal behaviors. If, after careful assessment, voice training is indicated, then future professional relationships should be planned with care.

3

Planning Behavioral Change in Voice Training

The purpose of voice training is to modify those behaviors responsible for vocal output that are judged to be unsatisfactory or inappropriate when compared to those behaviors that are judged to be "within normal limits." Many voice specialists have stated that these modifications are more of an art than a science, which may be true to some extent. However, the authors would argue that both clinician and client must pursue a process of change that is systematic, comprehensible, and productive in terms of achieving the goals of the training program.

The approaches used by clinicians vary from planning aimed directly at modifying specific motor behavior associated with the disorder to "wholistic" approaches that encompass broader or more general techniques of vocal improvement. Both the specific and wholistic approaches share much in common, for example, a comprehensive, sequential plan involving the clinician and client; a supplemental program of everyday management; evaluation; and counseling if indicated.

APPROACHES TO VOICE TRAINING

While all remedial programs have much in common, it is likewise true that not all clinicians approach voice modifications in the same way; much depends upon the philosophy, training, and experience of the individual. Training programs may be classified as either *wholistic* or *specific* in approach.

Wholistic Approaches

There are a number of voice training approaches that may be described as *wholistic* in their treatment of voice problems. The term wholistic is used to define any approach that deals with the broader, fundamental attributes of voice production, such as adequate breath support, easy, effortless phonation, pleasing quality, and responsiveness to the meaning and intent of communication. Wholistic approaches tend to become a complete voice program and often include drill on many aspects of vocal behavior. Indeed, there is the implicit assumption that a complete voice program is prophylactic and basic to the improvement of verbal behavior. Because the techniques used are broad, different types of voice problems are often treated in much the same manner.

The most widely used wholistic approach employs a full program of work with the basic processes of voice. The client learns to breathe, relax, initiate voice easily, resonate, and vary his voice in a systematic series of drills.[1] It is assumed that by the time the client has completed the prescribed program, the voice problem will be solved. A client may undergo breathing exercises even though his use of breath control for phonation appears adequate; he may be drilled on resonation exercises because the voice judged "good" is usually full or resonant. The use of singing exercises in voice training embraces much the same kind of philosophy.[2]

Other approaches to voice training that are classifiable as wholistic are the chewing method of voice rehabilitation and the use of systematic desensitization in stimulus situations, both of which differ markedly from the approach described above and cannot be appraised in the same manner. In the chewing method, for example, neither breathing nor relaxation drills per se are recommended, since the act of chewing itself is reported to be responsible for the restoration of these processes.[3] The client is asked to produce voice while chewing an imaginary morsel. According to the proponents of this method of voice rehabilitation, the physiological process of chewing does much to restore normal laryngeal valving.

The use of systematic desensitization in carefully constructed hierarchies of difficult voice situations is also classified as a broad or wholistic approach to voice rehabilitation.[4] This method of treatment addresses the day-to-day situations in which the greatest difficulty of voice usage occur. Training is not concerned with the manipulation of specific vocal behaviors in the clinic but rather with handling situations where vocal output is hampered by the presence of negative emotion in the client. The basic assumption underlying this therapy, of course, is that the client's voice problem will self-correct when he is able to free himself from the unwanted negative emotion.

The concept in voice training that there are many paths leading to the desired goal seems to be true, in part, because proponents of all methods

---

[1] Breathing, relaxation, phonation, resonation, and prosody procedures may be found in Chapters 6–10.

[2] The singing approach is discussed in Chapter 11.

[3] The chewing method is presented in Chapter 11.

[4] Systematic desensitization procedures are presented in Chapter 11.

report success for their clients with their special approach. It might even be true that the clinician (or client) succeeds in spite of the approach chosen. In the general improvement program, the singing approach, and the chewing method, the learning theory employed tends to remain unstated. Furthermore, as the clinician and client move from one phase of training to the next, goals shift and techniques of management are varied. Criteria for success appear to rest upon general rather than specific evidence. The claims for success for all wholistic approaches appear to be based on empirical rather than experimental evidence.

Specific Approaches

The specific approach to voice rehabilitation is defined as any attempt to identify and modify specific laryngeal or cavity behaviors judged inappropriate to terminal behaviors "within normal limits." A program of specific voice training necessarily includes the identification of the target behaviors to be modified in terms of their physioacoustic characteristics and a program designed to modify these behaviors to specified terminal behaviors.[5]

Since the target behaviors are clearly identified and studied in terms of both the physiological processes and acoustic results, the goals in training may be stated with precision and the criteria for success easily determined.

The specific approach avoids working systematically with any process of voice that is considered adequate, such as breathing or relaxation. Since the approach is concerned with specific behaviors, behavior modification techniques can be systematically applied.

Throughout the training program, the clinician must be concerned with shifting the client's laboratory control of voice to carry-over and maintenance of new behaviors in functional speech.

Whatever approach is selected, the clinician and client should abide by the general principles and sequence of the chosen method in order to maintain continuity and to eliminate confusion.

PLANNING THE TRAINING SEQUENCE

Almost all voice programs include at least four phases in the overall training sequence:

Phase I: Discussion, instruction, sensory training
Phase II: Modification of target behaviors, stabilizing control in the clinic, early attempts at stabilization elsewhere
Phase III: Strengthening new behaviors and decreasing the old behaviors, intensifying carry-over program
Phase IV: Terminal program and check-up

[5] Specific procedures for modifying laryngeal and cavity behaviors are presented in Chapters 4 and 5.

The difference between the phases is primarily one of emphasis. In Phase II, for example, work is concentrated on getting the client to produce the new behaviors and to strengthen them. In Phase III, the emphasis is upon getting the client to increase the use of the new behavior and suppress the use of old behavior both in the clinic and in day-to-day situations. It should be understood that instruction, discussion, and sensory training continue on from one phase to another.

As in all programs, the long-range goals need to be stated in behavioral terms. If these are stated in terms of "entering behaviors" and "terminal behaviors," the task of ordering the methods and materials of the program will become more explicit and precise. The entering behaviors are the physioacoustic processes that underlie the client's voice problem before training, and the terminal behaviors are the physioacoustic processes the client should possess after the training program is completed. All programs and phases of behavior management need to have goals stated in terms of the behaviors desired. The criteria governing success need to be stipulated in advance for each segment of planning.

Discussion

The clinician does more than present stimuli and handle the consequent events of the vocal response. He must serve as a teacher throughout all phases of clinical management.

The first phase of training is concerned with several steps, beginning with analyzing and discussing the client's voice problem in general. The clinician needs to ask such questions as "What's wrong with your voice?" or "What do you think is happening when you produce voice?" Basically, the clinician needs to teach his client to identify his problem, first in broad terms, then in very specific terms. The client needs to be taught what he is doing physiologically that is contributing to the voice problem.

Sensory Training

In order to accomplish the task of specifically identifying the underlying physiological processes that account for the voice problem, an extensive program of sensory training needs to be undertaken. The aim of this program is to teach the client to identify both the acoustic phenomena and physiological processes that deviate from the norm by means of a sensory program of auditory and kinesthetic discrimination.

GUIDELINES

1. *The clinician should be able to model a wide range of vocal outputs for his client.* The abilities of clinicians vary considerably. A clinician is at a disadvantage if he cannot present orally a stimulus that he wants the client to imitate. It is possible to use tape-recorded models or even a model who can supply the needed stimulus; however, either method can be in-

convenient. The question also arises as to whether a clinician with a basso voice should model voice for a client with a soprano voice. The problem, however, is not as great as being unable to model voice with any degree of accuracy at all. If a clinician has difficulty in modeling stimuli, he or she would be wise to practice extensively with professional help until able to perform satisfactorily.

2. *The client should be able to discriminate the acoustic phenomena associated with his problem as modeled by the clinician.* The models presented may be easy to identify at first and then should be made more difficult; that is, broad, then fine discriminations should be elicited.

3. *The client should be able to discriminate the acoustic phenomena associated with his problem as presented by tape-recorded samples of his own voice.* It is desirable to arrange these stimuli, if possible, in easy to more difficult presentations by carefully grading the samples.

Instruction

Before abnormal physiology can be discussed, the clinician should explain the processes of phonation to his client. Because of the complexity of the structure and function of the larynx, this type of instruction is not always an easy task. The authors recommend that a fairly simple yet clear-cut presentation be made. A detailed, academic presentation may not be necessary, for such a procedure is time-consuming and does not seem to promote any greater understanding or skill in handling vocal tasks successfully than does a more simplified presentation. Discussion should focus upon the nature of the vocal folds and how they function in normal speech, including the interrelationships between breath pressure, laryngeal valving, and resonance. The authors also favor discussion of the various parameters of voice when appropriate (e.g., quality, pitch, intensity, and time or duration).

Eventually, the instruction should focus on what the client is doing physiologically when he produces voice. It is important that he understand, even in a simplified version, the nature of the physiological processes that underlie the voice problem.

In explaining the processes involved in voice production, the clinician can make liberal use of models, diagrams, charts, illustrations, and frames from high-speed photography. These materials are usually better than self-made sketches and can serve as a permanent reference for the client. Furthermore, sketching takes time and requires skill, and often the sketches lack the detail necessary to tell the story vividly and accurately. Illustrations are abundantly available in standard texts and professional materials.

In summary, the preliminary training program should accomplish its goals of (a) answering some of the general questions concerning the nature of the client's voice problem, (b) teaching him to identify specifically the acoustic phenomena associated with the problem, (c) instructing him to understand the underlying physiological processes involved in his problem, and (d) setting the stage for self-correction and monitoring of his voice through a thorough program of instruction.

Modification of Target Behaviors

Modification of target behaviors begins very early in the training program and continues throughout all phases of the total program. The techniques used in working with a client should be aimed directly at changing the physiological processes responsible for the voice problem. Modification techniques typically include (a) instructing the client how to manage a given task, (b) demonstrating (modeling) the acoustic response wanted and asking him to echo it, and in some instances (c) manipulating the client's structures in order to produce the effect desired (e.g., manipulating the thyroid cartilage).

GUIDELINES

1. *The clinician should clearly identify the behavior to be changed in terms of its physiology.* The initial diagnostic session usually gives the clinician a lead as to the nature of the problem. Subsequent diagnostic probing develops further insight into the nature and extent of the deviant behavior. The tasks, then, that are selected to change the target behaviors should be directly related to the physiological processes involved.

2. *The prognosis for changing the target behaviors should be favorable.* It is discouraging and a waste of time to work with a client on a voice problem that has a poor prognosis. Before formal training begins, the clinician should spend some time in determining whether the client is capable of changing his voice problem toward more normal behavior. The authors recommend a period of diagnostic assessment in cases where the prognosis is in question.

3. *If there is more than one target behavior to modify, study each in terms of which should be approached first in program planning.* There are several points to remember when selecting one particular behavior to start with over another:

(a) Choose the behavior change that will give relief to the client and ease his concern.

(b) Choose the behavior that will yield most readily to training.

(c) Choose the behavior change that is needed before success can be achieved on another.

4. *The client should be able to discriminate between correct and incorrect trials of his own vocal output.* The program of kinesthetic and auditory discrimination should be continued throughout the training program. The client should not only be able to make fine discrimination of stimuli presented by the clinician, he should be able to discriminate between correct and incorrect trials of his own. For example, if the clinician models a

moderately breathy *ah* and asks the client to echo his response, the client should be able to know whether or not he has succeeded. This goal may be reached in two stages, first by the clinician signaling "correct" and "incorrect," and second by the client signaling "correct" and "incorrect" after he has produced the *ah*. One of the early goals of the clinician is to get the client to self-correct, for the client must be continually on the alert to maintain and strengthen the new behaviors and suppress the old. Self-correction should begin early in training and continue throughout all phases of the program. Self-correction usually develops as a direct consequence of a successful program of sensory training.

5. *The clinician must be highly analytical of the client's responses.* The successful management of the consequences following response is crucial in training, for the clinician must determine the next stimulus by the client's output. The clinician typically signals the client that his vocal output was "better," "same," or "worse" than before when being matched with a modeled stimulus or when asked to repeat an attempt. The clinician must decide what responses he will accept or reject; therefore, listening carefully to the response of the client becomes critical to the modification process. Eventually, the client must be able to monitor and identify his own attempts as "satisfactory" and "unsatisfactory"; therefore, the client must also develop keen insight into the nature of his responses.

6. *Teach the client how to contrast the new behavior with the old way of producing voice.* The principle of negative practice can be put to good use in voice training. After the client has stabilized his new behavior, have him produce voice "the old way." Contrast the new behavior with the old.

7. *The client should be taught to monitor his own voice in terms of sensory feedback systems.* The feeling as well as the acoustic feedback of voice production is vital to success. The client should concentrate upon the PTK of tone production, that is, the proprioceptive, tactile, and kinesthetic sensing of both satisfactory and unsatisfactory attempts to produce voice.

8. *In developing voice, move from easy to more difficult speech materials.* Good phonatory results achieved on any given step need to be applied to more difficult materials. A basic sequence used by many clinicians is the following: (a) low back vowels, (b) vowel-consonant combinations, (c) consonant-vowel combinations, (d) consonant-vowel-consonant combinations, (e) disyllabic words, (f) multisyllabic words, (g) phrases, (h) sentences, and (i) selected reading passages. Selected conversational materials usually follow this sequence.

9. *Length of training sessions should be adjusted to the client's needs.* Many clinicians ask, "How much time should be devoted to each session?" There is nothing sacred about half-hour, forty-minute, or one-hour sessions. Professional centers tend to schedule programs in blocks of 10, 12, 20, or more sessions of varying durations for purely financial reasons or scheduling convenience. One must not be a slave to these logistically contrived

patterns. During the early stages, more instruction (teaching) may be necessary than later when training settles down to routine behavioral procedures. Sessions, then, can be tailored to suit the client's needs, moving from forty-five minute sessions to twenty- or thirty-minute sessions or whatever is necessary to get the job done. It may be entirely possible (and likely) that a client with a hoarse voice simply cannot undergo more than ten minutes of manipulation without tiring. It would be folly to insist on forty-minute sessions with this type of client. The length of a session may also be adjusted to the behavioral changes that are taking place. If a client has been able to produce a given physiological process for the first time, it is wise to extend the session somewhat to insure control. If the clinician lays out his plan in terms of specific programs for all phases of the training program, he will be in a position to determine how long each segment will require. The rule, then, should be to apportion time to programs and goals, rather than to time blocks sold in terms of number and duration. One might judiciously plan the former to meet the convenience of the latter.

Stabilization

It is important for the clinician to achieve specific behavioral goals and to maintain control over newly acquired behaviors. In the clinic it is wise to spend time establishing the new behavior under a variety of conditions, ranging from easy to difficult. All too often the control of newly acquired behaviors gained in the training center dissipates quickly under the pressures of everyday life, and the older, unwanted forms reappear. Very often, additional behaviors appear quite suddenly. The clinician should strive to obtain many repetitions of the desired behavior in order to stabilize it.

Stabilization procedures start early in the clinical plan and continue throughout the program.

Carry-over

As in all behavior modification, the most difficult task is to get the client to perform successfully away from the clinic. The voice specialist should realize that many clients believe that training at the center alone will correct the problem and that carry-over to voice usage away from the clinic is automatic. Early in the training program the clinician must impress upon the client the fact that he must become his own master, and that all the success attained with the clinician will avail him little if he does not constantly monitor his vocal output outside the clinic.

Carry-over is a broad term and includes such concepts as (a) attempting to duplicate the goals achieved in the work at the center in a supplemental session away from the center, (b) performing successfully assigned tasks involving functional speech away from the center, and (c) monitoring vocal output in all oral communication.

Terminal Program

Training programs need to be concluded whether completely successful or not. If the goals of training have been clearly stated and criteria for success established and reached, termination need not present a major concern. One must not assume, however, that what the client can demonstrate readily in the clinic will carry-over to situations away from the clinic under pressure or tension. Terminal sessions are most generally concerned with maintaining successful voice usage away from the clinic. Planning strategies for outside performance and evaluating the results of these experiences should comprise much of the final sessions with the client. If the client has achieved continuing success, the intervals between sessions may be decreased until a termination date is agreed upon.

Check-up

Ideally, it would be good for the client to return for a voice check-up at intervals of thirty days, three months, six months, and one year. Realistically, clients rarely take the initiative to maintain such a rigorous follow-up program. If the modification program has been successful, the client will more than likely be content to let matters stand and not seek further evaluation of his voice. If he suffers regression, chances are that the clinician will hear about it, or somebody else will, possibly another voice specialist. The authors recommend that a thirty-day or three-month check-up be scheduled at the close of the formal training program and that a reminder be posted in the "tickler" file at the clinic.[6]

SUPPLEMENTAL CONSIDERATIONS

A comprehensive program should have several other inputs, in addition to the training sequence: (a) a program of periodic evaluation of progress; (b) a supplementary program of activities to be undertaken away from the training center, at home, work, and in the community; and (c) a program of counseling if indicated.

Evaluation

All programs should include evaluation checkpoints to determine progress, lack of adequate progress, or regression during given periods of work. Empirical data suggest that voice training is successful for a majority of cases. On the other hand, there are clients who can expect to achieve only limited gains, perhaps because of structural or functional defects that cannot be altered. There are also those clients who either cannot or are unable to

---

[6] Reminder cards may be filed in a month-by-month tickler file; as each month comes up, the receptionist calls the client to arrange an appointment.

change atypical vocal behaviors, and therefore routine vocal training is a waste of time. Often, this type of client can be helped by counseling in how to manage his atypical voice in the most effective manner in life situations.

The evaluation should take place in a specifically scheduled session. The diagnostic measures used to assess the problem initially can be used for the evaluation. Both clinician and client should take active part in the evaluation process. The materials used in the tape recording made at the first session can be tape-recorded again and compared. If the programs of Phase I have been structured and completed, a review of the goals, criteria for success, and the results should be analyzed carefully. After all of the data have been obtained and studied, the clinician and client should discuss the results in terms of achievement. If little progress is observable, the reasons should be sought and discussed.

Unfortunately, not all clients make satisfactory progress, even though the prognosis has been good and a rigorous program has been undertaken. If the client has failed to make progress, the clinician should modify his approach to the problem. He may also have to change the program of outside activities. It may be necessary to develop programs that will aid in shaping the behavior toward the desired goal more slowly; that is, more steps leading to a lower-level goal may be needed.

If a client continues in voice training and fails to succeed after all efforts have been made to develop a successful program, formal work must be terminated. After discussing fully the reasons for discontinuing direct training, the clinician and client should consider what can be done to manage the current vocal behavior more successfully in everyday life.

The Program of Outside Activities

Shortly after training begins, the clinician needs to institute a home-work-community program. This supplementary program may commence with the assignment of specific tasks to be practiced daily and culminate in an all-out attempt to strengthen the target behaviors in everyday experiences.

There are a number of compelling reasons why a supplementary program must be undertaken. The client must learn to become his own teacher and monitor. Furthermore, behavior is stabilized by rehearsal; therefore, the more new behaviors can be strengthened by repetition, the greater the probability that they will become habitual.

It is important that the client learn to execute each task successfully in the clinic in order to insure that he will not practice erroneously elsewhere. The clinician should rehearse the assigned tasks until perfection is gained.

The home-work-community program sets the stage for establishing functional use of new behaviors away from the clinician. If the client can perform target behaviors successfully in selected outside assignments, he should eventually be able to gain control in all his life situations.

The nature of the supplemental program may start with performance of short, specific tasks to gain control of a specific behavior (e.g., initiating voice with an aspirate attack). The assignment may be limited to a few minutes daily. It is better to have two short drill periods per day rather than one long period. With busy clients, you may suggest that a drill period be done in the car on the way to work, which assists in establishing a daily routine.

The work done by the client away from the center should be carefully monitored by the clinician. The client should demonstrate how he practices at home. He should be asked to record a session occasionally and bring the tape to the clinician for evaluation. Supplemental sessions can be lengthened as assignments change from vocalizing short syllables to more meaningful speech.

The supplemental program can be aimed at controlling the speaking environment. For example, a mother can be instructed to reduce the amount of general excitement at home for a child who has vocal nodules in order to curtail his vocal abuse. It is possible to better the environment, for example, by purchasing a humidifier to moisten dry air in winter, by filtering irritating allergens, or by eliminating sprays that are known to have a deleterious effect upon the voice.

A supplemental program can be prophylactic in nature and aimed at improving general health, hygiene, or eliminating undesirable habits such as smoking or excessive drinking. Gargling in the morning to reduce mucous or phlegm, getting more rest, and improving one's diet can improve general conditions that may aid voice production.

Finally, a supplemental program can be aimed at handling speaking situations more efficiently. The strategy of placement of auditors, the use of less overall intensity, the use of amplifiers for larger groups, and a host of other changes, can aid in improving how the client uses his voice in speaking situations.

Counseling

Very often, the diagnosis reveals that the client has an underlying emotional disturbance that is either directly or indirectly related to his voice problem. If the problem is serious enough to impede progress in the training program, a plan must be evolved for handling psychological counseling. The clinician has at least four courses of action he may pursue: (a) do nothing, (b) handle the counseling himself, (c) refer the client to a cooperating psychologist or psychiatrist and work with him, or (d) refer the client to another professional whose competencies better match the needs of the client.

To do nothing is to ignore the problem; and if the problem underlies the faulty vocal physiology, success in therapy is jeopardized. The voice specialist can only go as far as his formal training and ethics will allow. If the emotional problem of the client is beyond the ability of the clinician to handle properly, he should advise the client to seek psychological counseling, to be done in tandem with voice training. This type of referral is desirable, particularly if the counselor stays in close communication with the voice specialist. In a number of cases, the clinician may have to refer the patient for psychological counseling solely because of the nature of the emotional disturbance.

Speech clinicians often make the mistake of referring a client away without first trying voice training. One has no assurance that the client will either undergo counseling or psychotherapy, or that either of these processes will actually help the voice problem. Often, a transition period is needed to become more familiar with the client's problem before referral is considered.

4

Modifying Laryngeal Behaviors

The human larynx contributes a number of attributes to the acoustics of verbal communication. The following physiologies of the larynx are responsible for the certain aspects of speech function: (a) periodic vibration of the vocal folds, which can be sustained for varying lengths of time, resulting in relatively clear phonation; (b) variations in fundamental frequency, constituting a reasonable range potential; (c) on-off phonation, required by the sequence of code characteristics; (d) variations in amplitude of vibration, which permit intensity changes; and (e) partial valving, producing the voiceless vowels of whispered speech (i.e., the phoneme [h]).

Generally speaking, the disorders associated with laryngeal physiologies involve what is judged to be inappropriate or restricted use of the laryngeal sound-generating potentials, as well as decisions about their effectiveness. Disorders of laryngeal behaviors are presented in this chapter in terms of their physioacoustic properties, possible physiological bases, and common labels. Suggestions for modifying or changing these behaviors are given. It must be understood that the laryngeal behaviors described are all within the normal potential of individuals. They become problems when the effect of the behavior on the communication process is viewed by someone to be undesirable or to not meet the demands of the communication intent.

THE LARYNX AND VALVING

The valving of the larynx, especially of the vocal folds, is important not only to keep foreign matter out of the lungs and to aid in clearing them but also to provide a spectrum of sound potential for use in speech. Of course, no laryngeal wave form is produced at the extremes of valving (abducted and adducted), but, between these extremes, the varying degrees of valving participate in generating (a) the acoustics of laryngeal air turbulence (hypovalving) and (b) vibration of the vocal folds, the acoustics of optimal hypovalvular phonation and hypervalvular phonation. In addition, laryngeal valving is part of the production of the glottal plosive, which is associated with a number of disorders of speech.

Hypolaryngeal Valving

For the purposes of this text, the degrees of hypolaryngeal valving are (a) completely abducted; (b) partially valved; and (c) partially valved with vocal folds vibrating, or hypovalvular phonation.

Completely Abducted

PHYSIOACOUSTIC DESCRIPTION.   Vocal folds are in the completely abducted position and the larynx provides no valving. There is no resistance to airflow at the level of the larynx, so sound generation is confined to the modulation potentials of the supraglottal resonators, especially the oral cavity (buccal sound). Speech, therefore, consists of orally produced voiceless plosives, fricatives, and affricates, with little, if any, noticeable air turbulence associated with the cavity configurations for vowels, nasals, or glides. Extremely short phrases in connected speech are common, necessitating frequent renewal of air supply. If the larynx has been surgically removed and no air way exists between lungs and mouth, voiceless plosives, fricatives, and affricates must be produced by compression of local oral or pharyngeal air (buccal speech). Refer to the section on speech without a larynx near the end of this chapter for discussion of esophageal phonation and buccal speech.

POSSIBLE BASES.   Vocal fold paralysis (bilateral) in the completely abducted position; bilateral cordectomy; laryngectomy; myasthenia larynges and other similar conditions; conversion symptom.

COMMON LABELS.   Aphonia; abducted aphonia; hysterical aphonia; and the impairment labels noted above.

BEHAVIOR CHANGE INDICATED.   Provide laryngeal valving to the extent possible, even if only for whispered speech. If valving is unsatisfactory or impossible, establish a substitute vibrator (pseudo glottis).

PROCEDURES

1. Attempt any voluntary means that might produce laryngeal valving, especially those that are nonspeech oriented, like laughter, coughing, humming, or singing. This is particularly necessary if conversion symptom is suspect.

2. Occasionally, physical actions will help; for example, attempt laryngeal valving while lifting weights, pressing on table, pulling or pushing an object.
3. If no laryngeal valving or acoustic wave form can be generated, follow procedures for developing a pseudo vibrator, p. 47.

Partially Valved

PHYSIOACOUSTIC DESCRIPTION.   Vocal folds and the laryngeal valve are only partially abducted. Vocal folds are either held somewhat rigid or are far enough apart to not vibrate. The generated wave forms are the result of air eddying and whirling against the constricted surfaces. The amount of turbulence is a function of the degree of laryngeal constriction and the amount of airflow. This accounts for "loud" and "soft" whispers.

Speech consists of orally produced voiceless plosives, fricatives, and affricates produced orally, as noted above, and voiceless glides, nasals, and vowels [h] supplied principally by laryngeal turbulence exciting supraglottal cavity spaces. This is especially true for low vowels, since the oral resistance to airflow is minimal.

Phrases during speech are usually very short with frequent renewal of air supply. Renewal of air is often accompanied by stridor or gasping. Of course, whispering is appropriate to intimate situations where physical distance is not an obstacle to communication; it is perceived as a disorder when it is the only form of speech or occurs sporadically and unpredictably.

POSSIBLE BASES.   Vocal fold paralysis, unilateral or bilateral, in a partially valved position; cordectomy; myasthenia larynges; hysterical condition; learned behavior.

COMMON LABELS.   Whispering; aphonia; hysterical aphonia; conversion symptom of hysterical condition.

BEHAVIOR CHANGE INDICATED.   Increase laryngeal valving so that vocal folds are permitted to vibrate. Develop ability to sustain vocal fold vibration for code and paracode purposes.

PROCEDURES.   Refer to procedures for completely abducted behavior. Increase reservoir of air in lungs as a means of vibrating the vocal folds; pinch lamina plates of the thryoid cartilage as a means of approximating vocal folds.

Hypovalvular Phonation

PHYSIOACOUSTIC DESCRIPTION.   The vocal folds, although only partially valved, are able to vibrate. During the vibratory cycle the vocal folds move away from and toward each other and may not touch; hence, the closed phase is considerably shorter than the opening and closing phases.[1] This accounts for the noticeable air turbulence. The sound generated is a combination of two types of airstream modulation, namely, narrowed passage and vibrating structures.

The speech possesses a "breathy" quality. Phrases are short, but longer than in whispering. Vowels tend to be initiated with an aspirate attack. There is frequent renewal of air supply with possible gasping. The ends of phrases are often spoken on residual air. Delayed phonation after release of voiceless consonant [tʰeɪk] as in "take" is common, and frequent substitutions of voiceless allophones for voiced sounds occur, especially at the ends of phrases. Speech lacks loudness. Use of this quality often attracts comments of "shyness" and "timidity."

POSSIBLE BASES.   Laryngeal paralysis; myasthenia larynges; cordectomy; puffy, edematous vocal folds; excessive vocal strain; phonating at a fundamental frequency low in the range potential; learned behavior.

COMMON LABELS.   Husky; breathy; hypovalvular phonation; aspirate voice; inadequate loudness.

BEHAVIOR CHANGES INDICATED
1. Increase laryngeal resistance to the airflow during phonation.
2. Develop better control of air during exhalation for speech.
3. Work on improving the amplitude potential.
4. Shift the average fundamental frequency (modal pitch) if it is inappropriate.

PROCEDURES
1. Develop a greater reservoir of air, Chapter 8.
2. If the client uses thoracic breathing, modify to central control, Chapter 8.
3. Work on breath control for voice, Chapter 8.
4. Encourage phonation closer to the release of the voiceless consonants by reducing the number of voiceless consonants in phrases for sustaining better valving, Chapter 8.
5. Have client hypervalve the larynx, then release the airflow. Ask him to "sense" the feel of pinching the throat as he hypervalves.
6. After better phonation has been established, attempt to increase loudness, Chapter 6.
7. If the modal pitch is inappropriate, shift the average fundamental frequency to an optimum level, Chapter 6.
8. Increase the length of vowels in stressed syllables, Chapters 6 and 10.

[1] A complete cycle of optimal vibration is comprised of opening, closing, and closed phases. In this context, the closed phase is shorter in hypovalvular phonation than in optimal phonation.

9. If psychological counseling or medical treatment is indicated, make the necessary arrangements for it, if this is acceptable to the client.
10. If the usual techniques do not modify behavior toward more optimal laryngeal valving, and if medical or psychological help is not appropriate or acceptable to the client, focus on management of life situations to compensate for laryngeal hypovalving—that is, suggest the use of amplifying equipment; advise the client to avoid strain by utilizing more intimate speaking situations and by not speaking in high ambient noise, where possible. Vocal demands requiring loud talking should be avoided.

Hyperlaryngeal Valving

For the purposes of this text, the two degrees of hyperlaryngeal valving are (a) hypervalvular phonation and (b) completely adducted phonation (sporadic).

Hypervalvular Phonation

PHYSIOACOUSTIC DESCRIPTION. Vocal folds are pressed more tightly together during phonation, thereby increasing the length of the closed phase during the vibratory cycle, giving rise to greater laryngeal resistance to airflow. Phonation tends to be loud and penetrating, as in yelling, hence the words *metallic* and *strident* have been used. Frequent use of coup de glotte or hard attack (glottal shock) on initial vowels. Increased subglottal breath pressure. Frequent insertion of the glottal plosive between two vowels [siʔælɪs], as in "see Alice." Vocal folds slap each other vigorously, and consequently, prolonged speaking may produce laryngeal irritation, fatigue, and loss of voice. Hypervalving may introduce irregular vibratory motions of the vocal folds and surrounding structures. Stridor is often noticed on inhalation. The length of the voiceless phoneme is often reduced. Hypervalving also reduces the size of the laryngopharynx and produces a change of pharyngeal wall surface tension that contributes to the characteristically loud, penetrating, and metallic voice.

POSSIBLE BASES. Learned behavior; hypertension; speaking under pressure; hysterical condition; hearing loss; vocal abuse (excessive talking or strain, as in yelling or cheerleading); hyperactive; hyperkinetic; high intensity talking; demanding, aggressive personality.

COMMON LABELS. Strident; harsh; pinched throat; hypervalvular phonation; metallic.

BEHAVIOR CHANGES INDICATED
1. Reduce laryngeal hypervalving during phonation.
2. Decrease time of closed phase of vocal fold vibration. Work for more optimal valving, with hypovalving used as a contrast reference. Use

aspirate or simultaneous attack on initial vowels instead of coup de glotte.
3. Reduce amplitude and subglottal breath pressure. Relaxed speaking.

PROCEDURES

1. Yawn prior to phonation.
2. Work on relaxation procedures, Chapter 7.
3. Work on linking between consonants and vowels, between vowels and vowels within phrases, and longer breath groups when meaning permits (sustained resonance, Chapter 10).
4. Reduce intensity of phonation.
5. If the modal pitch is inappropriately high, lower it, Chapter 6.
6. Include drill materials that employ an abundance of voiceless sounds, Chapter 8, wastage of air.
7. As a means of hypovalving the larynx, increase the number of voiceless consonants in sentences.
8. See Chapter 9 for further procedures in the easy initiation of phonation.

Counseling should concern management of the voice throughout the day and should include (a) a more leisurely pace; (b) less hyperactivity and tension; (c) preventative measures to avoid further laryngeal strain; (d) management of environmental situations; (e) avoidance of situations that require loud talking or speaking in high ambient noise environments; and (f) increased periods of vocal rest throughout the day.

Completely Adducted Phonation (Sporadic)

PHYSIOACOUSTIC DESCRIPTION.   Laryngeal valve (true vocal folds and often ventricular folds) is completely closed prior to phonation. The vocal folds especially are pressed tightly together prior to phonation. The initiation of vibration requires considerable struggle. Speech is frequently interrupted by spasmlike adduction of the vocal folds causing moments of aphonia. Speech is staccato, with frequent glottal shocks and marked increase in subglottal air pressure. Vibration of vocal folds may be irregular.

POSSIBLE BASES.   Hysterical condition (conversion symptom); approach-avoidance behavior.

COMMON LABELS.   Adducted aphonia, spastic dysphonia, hysterical aphonia or dysphonia.

BEHAVIOR CHANGES INDICATED.   More optimal laryngeal valving. Psychological or psychiatric assistance.

PROCEDURES.   Refer to procedures for hypervalvular phonation and also for sporadic changes (below). Clinician must accept speech disorder on its face value and sincerely try to help client. Once rapport is established, every effort should be made to incorporate the special services of a psychologist or psychiatrist.

Sporadic Changes in Laryngeal Valving

PHYSIOACOUSTIC DESCRIPTION.   During phrases and sentences, the speaker's phonation alters unpredictably; most notable is on-off phonation unrelated to the voiced and voiceless phonemes. Fluctuations in valving may be from phonation to whisper or complete abduction or from phonation to adducted aphonia for brief periods of time. Also, a valvular tremor may appear during phonation.

POSSIBLE BASES.   Hysterical condition; psychosomatic condition; myasthenia larynges; on-off phonation following periods of excessive laryngeal strain; neurological disorder affecting laryngeal musculature; learned behavior; malingering.

COMMON LABELS.   Hysterical aphonia; sporadic phonation; spastic dysphonia (described under completely abducted phonation); unpredictable phonation.

BEHAVIOR CHANGE INDICATED.   Sustain optimal valving during phonation appropriate to the voiced characteristics of speech.

PROCEDURES

1. Initially, if the etiology apears to be hysteria, the clinician uses procedures that involve "tricking" the individual into sustained phonation, for example, distraction, laughter, coughing, and humming.
2. The clinician should encourage phonation for other than speech reasons at first while gaining rapport with the client.
3. Occasionally, it is desirable to accept a physiological explanation for the laryngeal disorder and teach phonation using a pseudo glottis in order to establish rapport and gain the confidence of the client.
4. Introduce a psychologist or psychiatrist into the treatment plan after understandable speech is achieved, and the client will accept the additional help. The speech clinician should gradually withdraw from the treatment program.
5. If the problem is based upon a physical impairment, medical intervention is indicated; following this, emphasis during training sessions should be on sustaining phonation—humming, holding vowels longer, and so on.

BEHAVIOR OF THE VIBRATOR

The vibration of the vocal folds contributes major dimensions to the acoustics of verbal communication and deserves the label "voice." For the purposes of this text, the physiology of vibration can best be described in terms of (a) frequency generation by the modes of oscillation, (b) amplitude, and (c) noise generation.

The Larynx and Frequency Generation

As the vocal folds are moved across the airstream and are free to vibrate, their oscillation generates a fundamental frequency. Variations in length, weight (mass), tension, and subglottal breath pressure produce a range of fundamental frequencies. The extent of the range differs from individual to individual. As mentioned in Chapter 1, three modes, or registers, of vocal fold vibration have been identified: full fold (normal), part fold, or falsetto, and syncopated, or fry. Each mode is capable of generating a range of fundamental frequencies. Although there are three modes of oscillation, each with a particular range, there is considerable overlapping of fundamental frequencies, as is diagrammed in Figure 1.2. Therefore, an individual is able to produce the same fundamental frequency in three modes of oscillation. Vibration at a more rapid rate is possible in part fold vibration than in full fold or syncopated vibration; a slower rate is possible in syncopated than in full fold or part fold. The combination of all the modes produces a total range of frequency available for vocalization of approximately two and a half to three octaves.

The disorders of frequency relate primarily to the inappropriate use of the part fold and syncopated modes of oscillation. Other common deviations, such as monopitch, modal pitch "too high" or "too low," and limited range use, are discussed in the section on pitch in Chapter 6.

Inappropriate Use of Falsetto

PHYSIOACOUSTIC DESCRIPTION.   Inability to use modes of oscillation other than part fold (falsetto); vibration confined to shortened vocal folds or their thin marginal edges (length versus mass); generation of high fundamental frequencies when compared to others of same age and sex; quality "thin" or lacking richness. Phonation can be effortless, even breathy, but stridor and hyperlaryngeal valving are often present, especially in cases of congenital or traumatic webbing. Relatively limited range use; often reduced amplitude in speaking, although considerable loudness can be achieved, as in screaming.

POSSIBLE BASES.   Laryngeal webbing (trauma, congenital); psychological factors; endocrinologic disturbances; delaying of voice change because of early adolescence; learned behavior; precocious pubescence.

COMMON LABELS.   Falsetto; juvenile voice; immature voice; eunuchoid voice (male).

BEHAVIOR CHANGE INDICATED.   Establish full fold vibration (normal) and stabilize its use.

PROCEDURES

1. Attempt a precipitous decrease from excessively high frequency, hoping to create a "break" into full fold vibration.
2. Attempt to maintain good relaxation while working with the client.
3. Have the client fry at the lowest frequency in the falsetto, then suddenly increase intensity with a chest pulse.
4. Have the client tilt head back as far as possible and phonate easily.
5. Press on the thyroid cartilage to shorten the vocal folds after phonation is initiated.
6. Have the client yodel, cough, hum, laugh, or grunt as an approach to initiate normal full fold vibration.

Inappropriate Use of Glottal Fry

PHYSIOACOUSTIC DESCRIPTION.   Excessive use of fry or syncopated modes of vocal-fold oscillation; a crackling, bubbling sound; vocal folds adducted; nominal subglottic breath pressure and minimal airflow; marginal edges of folds vibrate in a syncopated, double-vibrating manner; generally low frequency and low intensity; bubbling sound noticeable particularly at ends of phrases; voice deenergized and sounds tired, fatigued; can occur as the only means of phonation; range of frequency possible; voice lacks projection; often confused with hoarseness; often used as an indication of boredom or sophistication.

POSSIBLE BASES.   Learned behavior; myasthenia larynges; hypothyroid condition; may occur with vocal strain and fatigue; possibly associated with a laryngeal pathology such as a contact ulcer; projection of a vocal personality.

COMMON LABELS.   Glottal fry; fry; vocal fry; flutter.

BEHAVIOR CHANGE INDICATED.   Establish full fold vibration (normal) and stabilize its use.

PROCEDURES

1. Raise fundamental frequency of phonation.
2. Attempt to increase the loudness of the vocal output, Chapter 6.
3. Develop both a greater supply of air and airflow from the lungs, Chapter 8.
4. Hypovalve the larynx, using a breathy voice to get full fold vibration.
5. If unable to modify vocal behavior, make a medical referral.
6. Additional materials and procedures are presented in Chapter 6.

Inappropriate Shifts in Mode of Oscillation (Pitch Breaks)

PHYSIOACOUSTIC DESCRIPTION.   Sudden, sporadic, uncontrolled changes in mode of oscillation, usually accompanied by marked changes in fundamental frequency; shifts from normal to falsetto, falsetto to fry, or normal to fry; pitch breaks similar to yodel; may also include diplophonia (that is, two separate fundamental frequencies produced concurrently); often associated with a laryngeal pathology that weights the vocal folds unevenly; difficult to control and often unpredictable; commonly found during voice change in adolescent males.

POSSIBLE BASES.   Learned behavior; laryngeal pathology or partial paralysis; fatigue; neurological disorders such as cerebral palsy; lack of coordination due to rapid growth during early adolescence; hypertension.

COMMON LABEL.   Pitch breaks.

BEHAVIOR CHANGE INDICATED.   Stabilize use of one mode of oscillation.

PROCEDURES.   Sustain vowel or phonation in appropriate mode of oscillation; relaxation is desirable if pitch breaks accompany excessive muscular tension; hypovalve larynx and increase airflow from lungs.

Two Fundamental Frequencies (Diplophonia)

PHYSIOACOUSTIC DESCRIPTION.   A relatively rare phenomenon where two fundamental frequencies are produced simultaneously by the larynx. This may be due to the vocal folds vibrating segmentally at two fundamental frequencies or to a second vibrator, such as the ventricular folds, also vibrating. It may occur as an aspect of dysphonia when vocal folds are weighted unevenly by a pathology. It can be performed as a trick, especially when the two frequencies are in harmony.

POSSIBLE BASES.   Learned behavior; laryngeal pathology that weights vocal folds unevenly.

COMMON LABEL.   Diplophonia.

BEHAVIOR CHANGE INDICATED.   Establish use of one fundamental frequency during phonation.

PROCEDURES
1. Hypovalve the larynx if it is hypervalved, p. 76.
2. Use a yawn approach to phonation, Chapter 9.
3. Use a breathy approach to phonation, Chapter 9.
4. Decrease tension by relaxation procedures, Chapter 7.
5. Experiment with other fundamental frequencies (modal pitches), Chapter 6.
6. If the client is using too much force, reduce loudness.
7. Find a fundamental frequency level that does not have the two frequencies and stabilize it.

The Larynx and Amplitude

As mentioned in Chapter 1, the contribution of the larynx (specifically, the vocal folds) in producing sound energy differences (amplitude changes) is related to the degree of laryngeal valving, the mode of oscillation, the intrinsic tension of the vocal folds themselves, and the amount of subglottal air pressure or airflow. Maximum amplitude of the vibrator results from optimal valving, near the middle range of the normal mode of oscillation, with adequate intrinsic tension of the vocal folds and sufficient subglottal air pressure to achieve the amount of energy required. To vary any of these factors would alter the amplitude of vocal fold vibration. For example, hypovalving the larynx, increasing subglottal airflow, while holding a low fundamental frequency constant greatly reduces the amplitude and results in insufficient loudness to meet certain communication needs.

It should also be observed that changes in vocal energy have physical and psychological dimensions—the individual's perception of physical space and barriers to communication (ambient noise) and his perception of psychological space. Occasionally, the amount of energy used by a speaker is an indication of his feeling too close (weak phonation) or too far away (forceful phonation). Energy changes also make up one aspect of stress, or dominance of syllables and words.

It is difficult to document disorders of "loudness" because there are so many possible factors. Problems related to optimal use of amplitude in developing vocal skills are discussed in the section on force in Chapter 6. If the clinician's judgment is that the client uses insufficient loudness, the authors suggest a careful analysis of the other physiological variables to determine if vocal intensity might be improved by altering them.

The Larynx and Noise Generation

Laryngeal noise is the result of air turbulence associated with hypovalving, laryngeal hypervalving, and irregular vibration of the vocal folds or surrounding structures. In addition, laryngeal noise may possess unpredictable frequency shifts or pitch breaks. These possible sound sources produce a wide spectrum of laryngeal noise because different portions of each may be found in any one individual's sound composite. No two laryngeal noise phonations are exactly alike.

Laryngeal noise can be a learned as well as a pathologic behavior. It is often found with anger and yelling. Constant laryngeal noise is an indication of pathology. Experimental procedures may be utilized to ascertain if the pathology is responsible for the behavior.

PHYSIOACOUSTIC DESCRIPTION. Phonation aperiodic with proportions of air turbulence and laryngeal hypervalving contributing to harsh-strident effect; lack of clear tonal quality; phonation may have evidences of pitch breaks because of sudden changes in oscillation; struggle behavior to initiate phonation; phrases are often short because of excessive air flow through the larynx; marked use of the coup de glotte; stridor or gasping on inhalation; phonation may lack power or energy, with limited frequency range use; fundamental frequency often low in range potential.

POSSIBLE BASES.   Laryngeal pathology such as nodules, cysts, polyps, or carcinoma; puffy, edematous conditions; chronic laryngitis; myasthenia larynges; paralysis; endocrine changes; learned behavior.

COMMON LABELS.   Husky; hoarse; rough; disphonia; gravel throat; ventricular phonation.

BEHAVIOR CHANGE INDICATED.   Produce as clear phonation as possible for speech.

PROCEDURES
1. *Experimental procedures* should be utilized initially to determine if improved phonation is possible. These should include, but not be limited to, changes of fundamental frequency (usually higher); varying the degree of laryngeal valving (usually hypovalving); and altering the amount of airflow or subglottic breath pressure. If quality of phonation improves by manipulating variables such as these, prognosis is favorable and formal modification procedures should be established to stabilize the target phonation.
2. *Referral* is indicated if experimental procedures result in minimal or no improvement in phonation within a reasonable period of time, because no progress usually confirms a laryngeal pathology. Medical referral is strongly indicated. If hoarseness becomes progressively worse, medical referral is urgent.
3. *Management* involves direct attention to speaking in everyday situations, including vocal rationing in adverse speaking conditions and reduction of quantity of speaking. The use of the target phonation, determined under the experimental procedures, should be encouraged in ideal speaking circumstances. Total avoidance of loud talking, yelling, or shouting is strongly indicated to prevent continued misuse. The success with daily management is critical to the rehabilitation process.
4. *Specific procedures* used should be directed at curtailing vocal abuse by establishing contrasting behaviors of quietness or gentleness. Such techniques as soft, easy, breathy phonation, aspirate attack on initial vowels, relaxed attitudes in speech situations, avoidance of the coup de glotte, and stabilizing a more satisfactory fundamental frequency are all desirable. Silence for extended periods of time is not a speech procedure. Individuals who are hoarse must learn to drastically change their "vocal personality."

SPEECH WITHOUT A LARYNX

A number of distinguished publications have documented problems relating to the rehabilitation of the laryngectomee. The purpose of this text does not permit a detailed discussion of the impairment, surgical procedures, and alternatives to speech management. However, we will discuss advances in speech techniques that have been found to be beneficial.

The physioacoustic approach emphasized in this text suggests that the use of the term esophageal speech is inappropriate since buccal speech and esophageal speech would then appear to be different choices of rehabilitation. For example, the use of buccal speech has been discouraged because of the superiority of esophageal speech. Actually, a combination of these two types of speech is the most desirable approach. It would be better, therefore, to refer to the product of the pseudo vibrator as esophageal phonation, which provides the acoustic characteristics of the paracode and the phonation for the vowels, glides, and nasals. Esophageal phonation, then, is combined with buccal speech (oral compression of air) to produce the plosives, fricatives, and affricates that complete the speech signal.

Since intelligible speech after a laryngectomy demands the use of intraoral pressure to produce the voiceless phonemes, modification procedures should first aim to improve the buccal whispering of words and phrases such as *chicken soup* and *cheese cake*. Buccal whispering provides the basis for injection of air into the esophagus for the purpose of esophageal phonation.

Instead of speech interrupted to renew air supply, the laryngectomee should be taught to renew esophageal air as a function of the intraoral pressure on plosives, fricatives, and affricates. By means of this consonantal injection, the client is taught to inject the bolus of air into the esophagus simultaneously with the production of the voiceless consonants. For example, the intraoral pressure of the [tʃ] in *cheese* injects air into the esophagus for the [iz]. In the phrase *cup of coffee*, the [k] supplies the injected air for [ʌ], the [p] for [ʌv], the [k] and [ɔ], and the [f] for the [i]. Therefore, the entire phrase can be spoken without interruption. Longer phrases like "Joe took father's shoe bench out" provide abundant opportunities for consonantal injection without interrupting the flow of connected speech. Phrases that are composed of vowels, glides, and nasals ("We are alone now") should be avoided in initial lessons since they do not provide opportunities for consonantal injection.

Under ideal circumstances, consonantal injection is mastered in the first few speech sessions. Thereafter, procedures should concentrate on everyday words and phrases used by the client. The client should be encouraged to try to say anything in his daily routine. It is inappropriate to drill on nonsense syllables for they will delay acquisition of intelligible speech.

COMMON CLUSTERS OF LARYNGEAL EVENTS

We have been considering relatively discrete laryngeal events that may be associated with disorders. These discrete events are independent physiological variables, which can be combined with other variables to produce the laryngeal composite. Combinations have already been alluded to in the discussion of laryngeal noise. The possible combinations are perhaps endless, but the following deserve special mention.

Hyperlaryngeal Valving and Rapid Vocal Fold Vibration

The combination of hyperlaryngeal valving and high fundamental frequency is often indicative of laryngeal webbing. The phonation is penetrating or strident because of the effort involved in approximating the webbed vocal folds. The excessively fast rate of vocal fold vibration is the result of the shortened length of the vibrating surface. Often gasping will be noted on inhalation, and phonation at times will be difficult to initiate. If these behaviors cannot be modified, referral should be made to the medical profession.

Hypolaryngeal Valving and Slow Vocal Fold Vibration

The combination of hypolaryngeal valving and low fundamental frequency is a common laryngeal composite. The breathy, low pitch phonation has often been referred to as "husky" in the literature. In connected speech, a monopitch may also be noted. This tone composite alerts the clinician to the possibility of partial laryngeal paralysis or swollen, edematous vocal folds. Again, if behaviors cannot be modified, referral should be made to the laryngologist and the individual counseled with respect to management of voice in adverse speaking situations.

Frequently, altering the fundamental frequency (usually higher) will make possible better valving of the vocal folds. To produce frequencies low in the range potential usually necessitates hypolaryngeal valving. By asking the client to take an average frequency closer to the middle of the range, a less turbulent tonal quality can be realized.

5

Modifying Cavity Behaviors

The human resonating system, with its capability for adjustment, contributes certain basic attributes to verbal communication. The human resonating system should provide two airflow routes with cavities, openings, and couplings capable of producing the resonance characteristics of all of the phonemes that make up the code of any given language. The system, because of individual differences among speakers, also provides the dimension of voice quality unique to each speaker.

The vocal tract consists of two airflow routes, the pharyngo-oral air route and the pharyngo-nasal route. The first route depends on the velopharyngeal valve closing off the nasal passages, while the second depends on oral cavity serving as a cul-de-sac resonator to the main air tube.

CAVITY MODIFICATIONS
OF THE PHARYNGO-ORAL ROUTE

The changes in the tract configurations of the pharyngo-oral air system account for the characteristic resonances of all of the phonemes that make up the code, with the exception of the nasal consonants. The changes in the pharyngo-oral tract are determined by the position of the larynx, the tongue and jaw, the lips, the velum, and the contraction of the muscles of the pharynx.

The chief source of energy that excites the cavities is the wave form generated by laryngeal valving and vocal fold oscillation. However, the cavities may also be excited by the movement of air through narrowed orifices (fricatives) and by impounding and releasing the airflow (plosives). Changes in cavity dimensions, openings, and degree of coupling occur during the production of many consonants, as is true in the adjustments for glides and plosives. Vowels and continuants are characteristically more stable and do not change appreciably during production, exclusive of their on- and off-glides.

The many allophones of a given phoneme demonstrate that a speaker may utter a speech sound with varying adjustments of cavities and openings without losing the identity needed for the code. The paracode is also affected, as voice quality is perceptibly changed in the production of the different allophones of the same phoneme. The voice quality changes that occur, however, rarely interfere with the ability to decode the phoneme.

In the production of all non-nasal speech sounds, the pharyngo-oral route is used; therefore, an adequate seal by the velopharyngeal sphincter is required to eliminate excitation of the nasal passage cavities. The velopharyngeal valve plays an important role in human resonance, both with regard to the seal and timing of opening and closing on speech sounds.

The question often arises as to how tight the velopharyngeal valve must close to affect an adequate seal in the production of non-nasal speech sounds. A continuum of closures from adequate to totally inadequate seems to exist. Figure 5.1 illustrates that at least five degrees of closure are possible: (a) tight closure; (b) closure, but not tight; (c) near closure, with velopharyngeal valve opening less than opening to the anterior nares; (d)

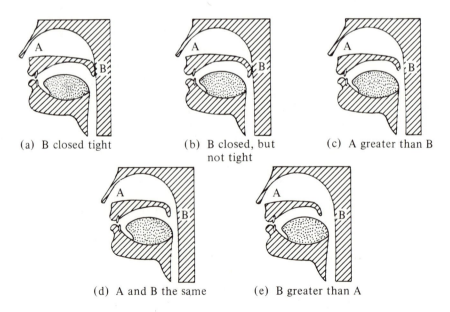

(a) B closed tight   (b) B closed, but   (c) A greater than B
                                  not tight

(d) A and B the same   (e) B greater than A

Figure 5.1
Five degrees of velopharyngeal closure. A = anterior nares; B = velopharyngeal valve.

velopharyngeal orifice the same as the anterior nares; and (e) velo-pharyngeal orifice greater than the anterior nares. It is possible for a skilled clinician to model extreme hypernasality, moderate hypernasality, slight hypernasality, and no hypernasality while producing the vowel [ɑ]. The mediating physiological process is unquestionably the differential adjustments of the velopharyngeal valve, yet the exact relationship between degree of opening and hypernasality has not been clearly established.

CAVITY MODIFICATIONS OF THE PHARYNGO-NASAL ROUTE

The changes that occur in the pharyngo-nasal route are chiefly concerned with the adjustments made in the cul-de-sac resonator, the oral cavity, in the production of the nasal consonants [m], [n], and [ŋ]. In order to produce the characteristic resonance of nasal consonants, the following requirements must be met: (a) airflow must be emitted from the nose only; (b) the pharyngeal cavity dimensions remain the same during production; (c) the velopharyngeal valve must be open; (d) the nasal passages must allow airflow without noticeable turbulence; (e) the oral cavity must be capable of being modified into three types of cul-de-sacs necessary for [m], [n], and [ŋ] (see Figure 5.2); and (f) the resonating system must be excited by the laryngeal generator. The differences between [m], [n], and [ŋ] in terms of resonance are the result of different sizes of the oral resonator.

TYPES OF CAVITY DISORDERS

There are two general types of resonance problems, based upon the adjustments of cavity sizes, shapes, couplings, openings, and textures. These are (a) voice disorders associated with cavity sizes and openings and (b) voice disorders associated with cavity coupling.

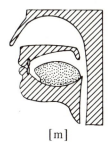
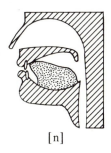
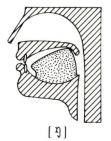

[m]   [n]   [ŋ]

Figure 5.2
Positions of tongue in oral cavity for [m], [n], and [ŋ].

Voice Disorders Associated with Cavity Sizes and Openings

Voice problems related to cavity sizes and openings may be classed in two groups: (a) high-frequency emphasis due to the use of small cavities and large openings and (b) low-frequency emphasis due to the use of large cavities and small openings.

Small Cavities and Large Openings

PHYSIOACOUSTIC DESCRIPTION.   The oral and pharyngeal cavities are decreased in size and the openings are increased. The tongue is postured high and forward in the mouth, increasing the opening between the pharynx and the oral cavity. The lips are spread wide on high front vowels but lack "pucker" on back vowels. The mouth is generally open wide on low vowels, but the tongue continues to be carried higher than optimal on all vowel positions, reducing the size of the oral resonator. The jaw is often forward when assuming these cavity adjustments. The thyroid cartilage may be raised, shortening the pharyngeal cavity. The soft palate is often elevated, increasing the opening between the pharynx and the oral cavity.

The acoustic characteristics related to a reduction in size of cavities and an increase in openings may be summarized as follows. The voice is perceived by the listener as higher than the fundamental frequency would indicate, chiefly because the energy in the higher formants is increased, while in the lower formants, the energy is decreased. The entire quality spectrum is shifted to higher frequency and greater intensity on the highs than is found in optimal resonance. The quality spectrum of consonants is similarly shifted, especially those requiring a reduced oral orifice (e.g., [s], [ʃ], and [θ]. The high front tongue position often gives rise to dentalization of the lingua-alveolar consonants. In cases where baby talk is employed purposely by females, a breathy quality may be heard. A male with a high resonance emphasis is often judged to be immature, lacking in strength, or weak. In cases where articulation and deportment are exaggerated and are coupled with high resonance emphasis, the person may be judged to be effeminate. A female is apt to be judged to be immature, lacking in vigor, or as younger than her actual age. As an adult, she may persist in using baby talk. If social interaction has been negative, the individual with high resonance emphasis may appear to be shy, withdrawing, or timid. On the other hand, the more effeminate type seems to enjoy his voice quality and may even exaggerate his speech style to suit his pleasure. Many females use infantile speech purposely in order to attract a member of the opposite sex or simply to call attention to themselves.

POSSIBLE BASES.   Learned behavior; small pharynx due to the absence of vertebrae; congenitally small cavities.

COMMON LABELS.   High frequency emphasis; thin, oral, immature, weak, effeminate, high-pitched voice; juvenile voice (when confused with falsetto); baby talk.

BEHAVIOR CHANGES INDICATED

1. Reduce the size of the openings of the oral cavity from pharynx and at the mandible.
2. Increase the size of the oral and pharyngeal cavities.
3. Work on articulation problems that remain, if any, after cavity size and openings have been adjusted.

PROCEDURES

1. Have the client posture his tongue farther back in the oral cavity, thereby reducing the size of the orifice from the pharynx.
2. Increase the size of the oral and pharyngeal cavities, pp. 167–169. Attempt to lower the thyroid cartilage, if it is raised unduly; manipulation by the fingers in a downward movement is often helpful.
3. Work on the concept of an open mouth and throat (megaphone effect); concentrate on the "feel" of the airflow moving through an unrestricted pharyngo-oral tract.
4. Contrast open positions with closed positions. Utilize the principle of negative practice.
5. Work on sustained resonance, pp. 169–171.
6. If an articulatory problem remains after high resonance emphasis has been modified, work on modifying the misarticulated sounds. If the lingua-alveolar consonants are dentalized, retract articulatory movements on these sounds to the alveolar ridge.
7. Consult Chapter 10 for additional procedures for developing resonance.

Large Cavities and Small Openings

PHYSIOACOUSTIC DESCRIPTION.   The oral and pharyngeal cavities are large in relation to the openings employed. The tongue is retracted, reducing the posterior oral orifice. The anterior opening to the oral cavity is small in relation to cavity sizes. The flow of air through the pharyngo-oral system is restricted. The thyroid cartilage is often lowered. The posture of the dorsum of the tongue, because of retraction, may impinge upon the larynx, reducing the efficiency of vocal fold vibration. In an effort to produce voice under these conditions, excessive muscular tension may develop in the lower pharyngeal area. Because of the increase in cavity size and decrease in openings, energy in the lower frequency formants is emphasized.

Acoustically, the voice is perceived as lower than the fundamental frequency would indicate. The increase in cavity dimensions, particularly the laryngopharynx, and the reduction in openings result in a voice that is perceived as being produced in the "back of the throat" and is described as "muffled" or "throaty." Voice quality is also judged as lacking in brilliance or clarity of tone. The person with low resonance emphasis may also have articulatory problems; that is, the quality spectrum is shifted to lower formant emphasis than is found in optimal voice production. Consonants often lack precision because of the resistance to airflow through the pharyngo-oral tract. The consonant [s], for example, is perceived as dull, and sounds requiring precision and pressure are often affected by airflow restriction. The person with low resonance emphasis has difficulty in projecting his voice and is often difficult to understand. Because voice quality is often judged as unpleasant, the client may suffer embarrassment and become shy and withdrawn.

POSSIBLE BASES.   Learned behavior; cerebral palsy; other neurological disorders or a neuromuscular condition; accidents causing such a condition; deafness, both total and severe.

COMMON LABELS.   Low resonance emphasis; throaty, muffled, guttural voice; backward placement; retracted voice; mushy.

BEHAVIOR CHANGES INDICATED
1. Increase the size of the openings by moving the tongue forward and opening the mouth.
2. Decrease the size of cavities in the pharyngo-oral tract.

PROCEDURES
1. Increase the openings in the pharyngo-oral airflow tract by (a) increasing the anterior opening of the oral cavity, pp. 168–169, and (b) having the client posture his tongue farther forward in the oral cavity, increasing the size of the pharyngo-oral orifice. Have the client put the tip of his tongue behind and touching the lower front teeth for vowels.
2. Reduce the size of the laryngopharynx by directing the client to raise his thyroid cartilage while phonating.
3. Work on the concept of frontal placement, Chapter 10.
4. Develop the concept of moving the airflow easily through the pharyngo-oral tract. Concentrate on the "feel" of airflow movement.
5. Work on relaxation in the lower pharynx and larynx in cases that exhibit excessive tension, Chapter 7.
6. Work on sustained resonance, Chapter 10.
7. Consult Chapter 10 for additional procedures for developing resonance.

Voice Disorders Associated with Cavity Coupling
Voice disorders associated with inappropriate cavity coupling may be conceived as occurring along a continuum between the two extremes of (a) positive nasal coupling, where the nasal passages are constantly coupled

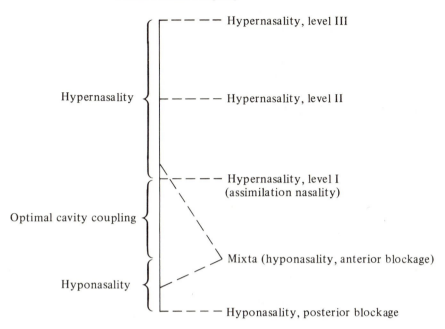

Figure 5.3
Continuum of nasality.

with the pharyngo-oral air tract; and (b) negative nasal coupling, where the nasal passages are never coupled with the pharyngo-oral air system. Optimal cavity coupling, where no problems of code or paracode may be perceived, occurs between the two extremes of positive and negative coupling. Nasality, then, may be described as a deviation from optimal cavity coupling in a direction toward either of the two extremes of constant coupling (hypernasality) or no coupling (hyponasality).[1] Figure 5.3 illustrates this continuum of nasality.

Voice disorders associated with positive nasal coupling occur when the nasal passages are (a) coupled on vowels adjacent to nasal consonants—partial hypernasality, level I;[2] (b) coupled on vowels and glides regardless of adjacent nasal consonants—constant hypernasality, level II; and (c) coupled at all times during speech—constant hypernasality, level III.

Voice disorders associated with negative nasal coupling are discussed in this text in terms of (a) *mixta*, or hyponasality with anterior blockage of

[1] Nasality as used in this text includes both hypernasality and hyponasality.
[2] Commonly referred to as assimilation or similitude nasality.

the nasal passages (i.e., nasal passages are positively coupled to the pharyngo-oral airflow route) and (b) hyponasality with posterior blockage and negative nasal cavity coupling.

Optimal Cavity Coupling

Between the two extremes in Figure 5.3, nasal coupling can be employed in an optimal manner; that is, there is a point on the continuum where non-nasal sounds are not perceived as hypernasal because of an adequate closure of the velopharyngeal sphincter, and nasal consonants are appropriately produced by the positive coupling of the nasal passages with the pharyngo-oral air route. The airflow in the latter instance is through the nose, as the oral cavity airflow route is blocked and functions as a cul-de-sac resonator. Velopharyngeal valving is appropriate to all phonemes and phonemic combinations in the sequencing of speech.

Positive Nasal Coupling

Partial Hypernasality, Level I

PHYSIOACOUSTIC DESCRIPTION.   The timing of the velopharyngeal seal is often delayed or anticipated on phonemes that precede or follow nasal consonants, and hypernasality occurs on the non-nasal sounds. If the velopharyngeal valve is permitted to open during the production of a non-nasal sound or sounds before a nasal consonant, as in *on, am, only,* the nasal passages are coupled with the pharyngo-oral tract and hypernasality results. If hypernasality occurs on non-nasal sounds before the nasal, the term progressive assimilation nasality is used.

Hypernasality on a non-nasal sound may also occur if the velopharyngeal seal is made too late following a nasal, that is, remains open after the non-nasal sound is articulated, as in words like *me, mate, next.* When the timing of closure is faulty on nasal–non-nasal combinations, the term regressive assimilation nasality is often used.

The problem may vary in severity from occasional to constant assimilation nasality, depending on the number of nasal phonemes in the speech signal. Greatest difficulty in timing the seal occurs when non-nasal sounds both follow and precede nasal consonants, as in words like *men, name, happening, mean, mint.* Assimilation nasality is a *partial* problem of faulty positive coupling; therefore, non-nasal sounds that are not adjacent to nasals are usually not affected.

POSSIBLE BASES.   Learned behavior; possible muscular incoordination.

COMMON LABELS.   Assimilation nasality; similitude nasality; progressive assimilation nasality; regressive assimilation nasality; whining speech; other labels when combined with laryngeal hypervalving.

BEHAVIOR CHANGES INDICATED

1. Develop appropriate timing of the velopharyngeal closure on (a) non-nasal sounds preceding nasals; (b) non-nasal sounds following nasals, and (c) non-nasal sounds between nasal consonants.
2. Lengthen vowel duration in cases where it is short to permit better timing and articulation in the coupling-uncoupling function.

PROCEDURES

1. Discuss the nature of assimilation nasality with the client. Use diagrams and other visual aids to illustrate the nature of the problem.
2. Provide a complete program of sensory awareness or discrimination, including auditory, visual, and kinesthetic systems, Chapter 10.
3. Establish a base line of success on non-nasal materials, Chapter 10.
4. Initiate vowels with a yawn to establish non-nasal production, then initiate the nasals.
5. Monitor nasal–non-nasal production by feeling the nose.
6. Work on vowel–nasal speech sound combinations, Chapter 10.
7. Work on nasal–vowel speech sound combinations, Chapter 10.
8. Work on vowel–nasal–vowel and nasal–vowel–nasal combinations, Chapter 10.
9. Stabilize control in words, phrases, and sentences, Chapter 10.
10. Contrast nasal and non-nasal speech sound production, Chapter 10.
11. Stabilize new behaviors in all speaking situations.

Constant Hypernasality, Level II

PHYSIOACOUSTIC DESCRIPTION.   The velopharyngeal sphincter is open, coupling the nasal passages with the pharyngo-oral air tract on vowels and glides. The opening at the anterior nares is equal to or less than the opening of the velopharyngeal sphincter; therefore, the nasal passages do not function as a cul-de-sac resonator. The position of the tongue on high front and high back vowels increases the resistance of the airflow through the mouth, increasing the airflow through the nasal passages—the line of least resistance (see Figure 5.4). Because the velum is positioned close to closure on non-nasal sounds, a *pneumatic* seal instead of a completely *neuromuscular* seal is made on those consonants requiring an increase in intraoral breath pressure (i.e., plosives, fricatives, and affricates). For example, in producing a plosive, the velum is "pushed" from its nearly closed position to a closed position, affecting a pneumatic seal sufficient for implosion; the velum is released on explosion as air pressure drops quickly in the oropharynx. In this type of constant hypernasality, the degree of hypernasality may vary as a function of degree of closure and cavity sizes. The chief acoustic effect is the hypernasalization of vowels and glides. The

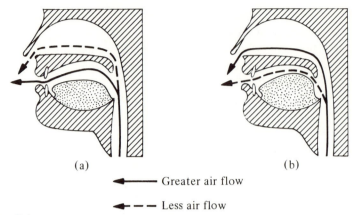

(a)   (b)

◄——— Greater air flow

◄— — — Less air flow

Figure 5.4
Varying resistance to airflow. (a) Airflow resistance through mouth is less.
(b) Airflow resistance through mouth is greater.

degree of hypernasality on given vowels and glides varies because of the
air pressure differential between the two air routes. This may be summarized
as follows: (a) High front and back vowels increase airflow resistance
through the pharyngo-oral tract, increasing the likelihood of nasal airflow
emission; (b) the oral cavity is less restricted on low vowels; hence,
resistance to airflow is less, decreasing the likelihood of nasal emission;
and (c) glides require changes in tongue position during production (i.e.,
from high to low, low to high); therefore, resistance to airflow will vary
with cavity size and opening.

POSSIBLE BASES.   Neuromuscular condition involving the velopharyngeal
sphincter; mild insufficiencies; short velum; submucous cleft of velum;
learned behavior.

COMMON LABELS.   Constant hypernasality, level II; nasality; hypernasality;
rhinolalia aperta; nasal speech; positive nasality.

BEHAVIOR CHANGES INDICATED
1. Develop an appropriate velopharyngeal closure for vowels and glides.
2. Reduce pharyngo-oral air tract resistance on non-nasal sounds by cavity
   adjustments.
3. Develop neuromuscular control of the velopharyngeal sphincter for
   plosives, fricatives, and affricates.

PROCEDURES
1. Determine the degree of velopharyngeal competency by diagnostic
   therapy, Chapter 10.
   (a) If the client is capable of making an adequate neuromuscular

closure, a full program of behavioral modification should be undertaken.

(b) If the client is *not* capable of effecting an adequate closure, concentrate on compensatory behavioral changes that will decrease
the problem (e.g., lowering and moving tongue forward to reduce
resistance, decreasing the amount of hypernasality).

2. Explain and discuss the nature of the problem with the client, using
visual and auditory aids.
3. Undertake a program of sensory awareness or discrimination, including
auditory, visual, and kinesthetic systems, Chapter 10.
4. Develop a more effective neuromuscular closure of the velopharyngeal
valve by working on velar drills, Chapter 10.
5. Establish a base line of success on non-nasal materials, Chapter 10.
6. Develop a program leading from easy to difficult materials:
    (a) Base-line materials, easiest to produce.
    (b) Materials stressing high back vowels, then high front vowels.
    (c) Materials with nasal and non-nasal combinations.
    (d) Materials combining all levels of difficulty in words, phrases, sen-
    tences, and impromptu speech. Stabilize control.
7. Attempt to reduce resistance of airflow on high vowels by experiment-
ing with cavity adjustments.
8. Attempt to increase neuromuscular control on plosives, fricatives, and
affricates.

Constant Hypernasality, Level III

PHYSIOACOUSTIC DESCRIPTION.   The nasal passages are constantly coupled
with the pharyngo-oral air system on all speech sounds. The velopharyngeal
sphincter is unable to affect an adequate seal on consonants requiring pressure or is inoperative altogether. The nostrils are often "pinched" to assist
in occluding the nasal passages on non-nasal speech sounds. The two air
tracts are merged on the production of all speech sounds. Voiced plosives
are modified in the direction of nasal consonants. Because the opening
between air tracts is often large, resonance on vowels and glides can be
described not only as constantly hypernasal but "muffled" as well. As the
airflow is increased through the nasal passages on plosives, fricatives, and
affricates, turbulence is increased and is often heard as a nasal "snort." A
glottal plosive is often substituted for consonants requiring pressure build-
up. Inasmuch as many phonemes cannot be recognized, the code is greatly
affected and intelligibility is reduced. The voice and articulation problem
varies in degree of severity.

POSSIBLE BASES.   Neuromuscular deficit affecting the velopharyngeal seal;
cleft palate; submucous cleft; short velum; velopharyngeal sphincter fails to

function following surgery; paralysis affecting the sphincter muscles; possibly also a learned behavior.

COMMON LABELS.   Constant hypernasality, level III; nasality; hypernasality; rhinolalia aperta; cleft palate speech.

BEHAVIOR CHANGES INDICATED

1. Develop an adequate seal between the two air tracts, if possible.
2. Modify all compensatory behaviors, if optimal speech sound production is possible.
3. If optimal speech sound production is not possible, then (a) modify behavior to highest level of attainment; or (b) teach compensatory behaviors.

PROCEDURES

1. Determine the ability of the client to make an appropriate seal. If he cannot, discuss the alternatives available to him:
    (a) Medical referral to determine the feasibility of surgery.
    (b) The use of a prosthesis.
    (c) Clinical management after (a) or (b) has been undertaken.
    (d) Teaching compensatory movements only.
    (e) No further action.
2. Discuss the nature of the problem and initiate a program of discrimination.
3. Attempt to achieve an adequate seal between the two air tracts.
4. Concentrate on directing the airflow out of the mouth. Tell the client to monitor airflow by kinesthesis.
5. Develop a base line of success on non-nasal materials. Use the easiest-to-produce vowel and consonant combinations.
6. Increase the difficulty of the non-nasal materials.
7. Develop appropriate timing of the seal, combining nasal and non-nasal materials.
8. Materials and procedures are to be found in Chapter 10.

Negative Nasal Coupling

Hyponasality, Posterior Blockage

PHYSIOACOUSTIC DESCRIPTION.   The nasal passages are blocked posteriorly and cease to function as resonators on [m], [n], and [ŋ]. As a result of the posterior blockage, the nasal passages cannot function as part of the main resonating tube (see Figure 5.5). The oral cavity no longer functions as a cul-de-sac resonator for the pharyngo-nasal air tract but instead forms part of the main resonating tube, as the airflow emits from the mouth rather than the nose on nasal consonants. Acoustically, [m], [n], and [ŋ] are heard as

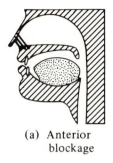

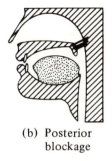

(a) Anterior
blockage

(b) Posterior
blockage

Figure 5.5
Hyponasality. (a) Anterior blockage. (b) Posterior blockage.

modified versions of [b], [d], and [g]. The voice quality is perceived as muffled in direct ratio to the number of nasal consonants in the speech sample. The client with a voice problem based on negative nasal coupling occasionally has difficulty in being understood.

POSSIBLE BASES.   Enlarged adenoids (in children); growths that block the nasal passages; allergies or colds, resulting in edema or secretions that block the passages; scar tissue because of surgery; congenital malformations.

COMMON LABELS.   Hyponasality; rhinolalia clausa posterior; nasality; "cold-in-the-head" speech.

BEHAVIOR CHANGES INDICATED.   No behavioral changes can be made until the condition is corrected. A medical referral should be made to determine whether or not the blockage can or should be removed. If the blockage is removed and hypernasality results, treatment may be necessary. Caution: If the velum is short and a seal has been possible because of the presence of adenoids, removal of the adenoids may result in constant hypernasality, level III. Surgery in this instance will have created a far greater voice and speech problem than existed before the operation. A careful assessment of the velum and the obstruction must be made by the speech pathologist and the surgeon before surgical intervention is recommended in borderline cases.

PROCEDURES.   If hypernasality results after surgery, follow the procedures recommended in constant hypernasality, levels II and III.

Mixta

PHYSIOACOUSTIC DESCRIPTION.   The nasal passages are blocked anteriorly and the velopharyngeal valve is unable to affect a seal or is inoperative. Thus, a *mixta* type of problem emerges—that is, positive nasal coupling on non-nasal sounds and negative nasal coupling on nasal sounds. Since the blockage occurs anteriorly, the nasopharynx and at least part of the nasal passages serve as a cul-de-sac resonator, as is illustrated in Figure 5.5a. The airflow follows the pharyngo-oral air route on both nasal and non-nasal speech sounds. If the velopharyngeal seal is incompetent at all times, the optimal resonance of the pharyngo-oral air tract is modified by the addition of a cul-de-sac resonator on the voiced components of sounds, and a characteristic muffled quality is heard. If the seal is competent, only nasal consonants will be affected. The [m], [n], and [ŋ] tend to be pressure release modifications of [b], [d], and [g], respectively, as the cul-de-sac permits an abbreviated nasalized antecedent to the release of the airflow on nasals. If the velopharyngeal valve is completely inoperative, the *mixta* problem is much more pronounced. Because of the muffled quality and the compensatory articulatory movements for [m], [n], and [ŋ] and adjacent sounds, the person with a *mixta* problem has difficulty in being understood.

POSSIBLE BASES.   Malformations, growths, or scar tissue that block the anterior portion of the nasal vault but do not occlude the vault as a whole; congenital insufficiencies of the velum.

COMMON LABELS.   Hyponasality; rhinolalia clausa anterior; *mixta*; "cold-in-the-head" speech; muffled speech; positive and negative nasal coupling; nasality. Misnomers: "talking through nose," nasal twang.

BEHAVIOR CHANGES INDICATED
After anterior blockage has been corrected:

1. Establish airflow through the nasal passages on nasal consonants.
2. If the velopharyngeal valve is inadequate but is capable of making a seal, or if the velopharyngeal valve is merely inactive, develop appropriate sealing for speech.

PROCEDURES
1. Develop velopharyngeal sphincter action, Chapter 10.
2. Direct airflow through the nasal passages.
3. Develop proper timing of the seal on nasal and non-nasal speech sounds, Chapter 10.
4. Also see the procedures for constant hypernasality, levels II and III.

6

Prosody

The assessment of a client's voice should include a systematic study of all of the parameters of voice, including pitch, rate,[1] and force,[2] as well as quality. The focus of attention in the voice disorders discussed in Chapters 4 and 5 was upon inappropriate quality and the underlying physiological processes involved, with emphasis on pitch and force. During the early stages of voice training, clinicians give instructions for handling pitch, rate, and force, while concentrating primarily upon modifying quality. However, clinicians do not characteristically treat pitch, rate, and force separately, except on some notable occasions, as when modifying juvenile voice. If a client demonstrates an inability to utilize vocal variety in speech, a program of training in the area of prosody should be considered.

Vocal variety is a requisite for effective communication, as meaning and emotion are conveyed by prosody as well as by the words one selects. Lack of vocal variety not only gives rise to monotony but well may be one of the contributing causes to the client's voice problem, as when a client uses only one level of intensity, or has a rapid delivery, or a pitch monotone that taxes vocal endurance. Normal voice production makes liberal use of varying all of the parameters of voice. It would seem wise, then, that some consideration be given to developing greater vocal variety in those clients who persist in using monotonous voice production after suitable vocal quality has been achieved. Usually, concentration in this area of work is best undertaken in the middle or closing stages of the training program.

---

[1] Rate as used in this text refers to duration of phonemic utterance as well as rate per unit of speech (i.e., syllables, words, phrases, sentences).

[2] Force as used in this text refers to use of all levels of intensity as well as changes in intensity on syllables, words, phrases, and sentences.

Vocal variety is concerned with the efficacious, simultaneous use of all of the parameters of voice. Prosody problems, however, may be more centrally concerned with one parameter than another; therefore, in this chapter, each parameter is presented separately. The clinician should keep in mind that there is a constant dynamic relationship, dictated by meaning and emotion, between quality, pitch, rate, and force. A systematic study of prosody gives the client an excellent opportunity to demonstrate his control over the physiological processes he has studied in isolation. In short, it gives him a chance to "put it all together."

It is not mandatory to follow the order of presentation in this chapter, as each of the parameters of voice can be studied independently or in any sequence that is consistent with good planning.

PITCH

The average person relies upon pitch changes to express his thoughts and emotions. Pitch change is one of the chief means by which we convey meaning and shades of meaning. While it is true that pitch is chiefly an instrument of expressing our thoughts, it plays an important role in revealing our emotions to others. For example, if an individual is happy, his pitch patterns are apt to cover a wide range, are slightly higher in modal level than usual, and are varied; if a person is unhappy or sad, the patterns are apt to be narrow in range, lower in modal pitch than usual, and less varied.

Voice Problems Associated with Pitch

People vary in their use of pitch, as some utilize it to maximum efficiency, while others do not. Many persons do not use pitch adequately, and some use it inappropriately. Several voice problems may be specifically related to the use of pitch. One group of these problems is related to something the client does that is not appropriate; for example, he uses too high modal pitch. Another group is related to the client's failure to use pitch effectively; for example, speaks on a monotone. The first group of problems needs to be handled by modifying the old behavior, while the second group requires a program of instruction aimed at acquiring new behaviors. The voice problems associated with pitch usage may be summarized as follows:

1. Use of too high or too low modal pitch level, including vocal fry.
2. Use of a narrow or restricted pitch range.
3. Use of part fold vibration and an inappropriate modal level, as in juvenile voice.
4. Pitch breaks.
5. Use of pitch monotone.
6. Use of monotonous pitch contours.

OPTIMUM PITCH

Most voice clinicians embrace the concept of optimum pitch, even though tests or measures to obtain this ideal pitch level have questionable validity and reliability. Supporters of the concept of optimum pitch postulate that every speaker has a pitch level within his range that is ideal for habitual use in formulating the majority of his pitch contours. This level is said to be the "most natural," the "most comfortable," the "one most easily resonated for the amount of effort expended," the most "full and rich," and so forth. Voice theorists further infer that optimum pitch is determined by the size, shape, and construction of the resonators (including the trachea), as well as by the length, thickness, tension, and density of the vocal folds. Inasmuch as humans vary with regard to these factors, optimum pitch must be determined for every individual. Refer also to Chapter 1 for additional information.

Most authorities agree that the average speaker has approximately two octaves of fully supported tones in his pitch range (not including falsetto). The optimum pitch level is described by some theorists as usually about one-fourth the way up from the lowest supported tone in the pitch range (including falsetto) and embracing as much as three half-tones (on the chromatic scale) at this level. Other theorists have been more concerned with stipulating the optimum pitch level as the place in the pitch range where the voice noticeably becomes "richer and fuller" for the amount of effort expended, or where a demonstrable difference in intensity can be observed when vocal effort is held constant, as indicated by West's manometric flame test.

Because the optimum pitch concept is tentative in nature, the clinician should weigh the facts involved carefully and determine what course he wishes to pursue with his clients. The authors feel that an attempt should be made to determine whether or not his client is using the best level for his voice. He does not feel that the clinician should *routinely* place the voice of his client at a level one-fourth the way up from the bottom of his total pitch range, despite the fact that this method may prove quite useful for many of his clients. Because many clients are either tone deaf, unable to sing, or do not have the ability to manipulate their voices properly in pitch range exercises, it may be both necessary and desirable to experiment with other methods of determining the "best level" for habitual use.

Determining Optimum Pitch

Several methods are currently used to determine optimum pitch. Select the procedure that seems to be best for the client. If a person is unable to sing a scale, the clinician must attempt to have him inflect his voice up the scale as far as he can go, including falsetto. Locate the highest note inflected with a pitch pipe or piano. If the client has difficulty in inflecting his voice, help him by modeling what you want. After you have located the highest note in his range, have him inflect his voice as far down the scale as he can manage and locate that pitch level with the aid of a pitch pipe. The determination of optimum pitch can then follow a standard procedure as soon as the two extremes in the client's range have been determined.

For those who are able to follow a diatonic scale (*do, re, mi,* etc.), the singing methods of locating optimum pitch may be used.

PROCEDURES FOR DETERMINING OPTIMUM PITCH BY SINGING

1. Whole-note calculation method:
   (a) Locate C with a pitch pipe or piano; use C_4 (262 cps) for women and C_3 (131 cps) for men. Normally, using C_3 and C_4 will start the subject at a pitch level that is in the lower half of his range.
   (b) Have the client sing as far up the scale as he can go, including falsetto. Use the Optimum Pitch-Location Chart (Figure 6.1) to assist you in relating the notes sung to the piano keyboard. (An example of this method of locating optimum pitch is presented in the Optimum Pitch-Location Chart to the *right* of Column III.)
   (c) Mark the last note sung in falsetto opposite the appropriate place in the chart. If the client has difficulty in singing the scale properly, model it for him, then sing with him to assist him in reaching the high note.
   (d) Return to C_3 (or C_4) and have the client sing down the scale, *do, ti, la, sol, fa,* etc., to the lowest note he is able to sustain. Be sure he follows the appropriate pitch levels for each note sung. Use the location chart (Figure 6.1) to follow the notes sung.
   (e) Mark the last supported note sung. Do not accept a note sung with glottal fry alone.
   (f) Locate the highest note sung in Column II and convert it into the corresponding whole notes indicated in Column III.
   (g) Locate the lowest note sung in Column II and convert it into the number of whole notes indicated in Column III opposite that level.
   (h) Add the number of whole notes derived in Steps f and g.
   (i) Divide the total number of whole notes by 4. The product represents the number of whole notes in one-fourth of the client's range.

Figure 6.1 ▶

Optimum pitch-location chart. A client who vocalizes *up* the scale from C_3 to C_5 (including falsetto) and vocalizes *down* the scale from C_3 to E_2 has a total range of 32 half notes, or 16 whole notes.

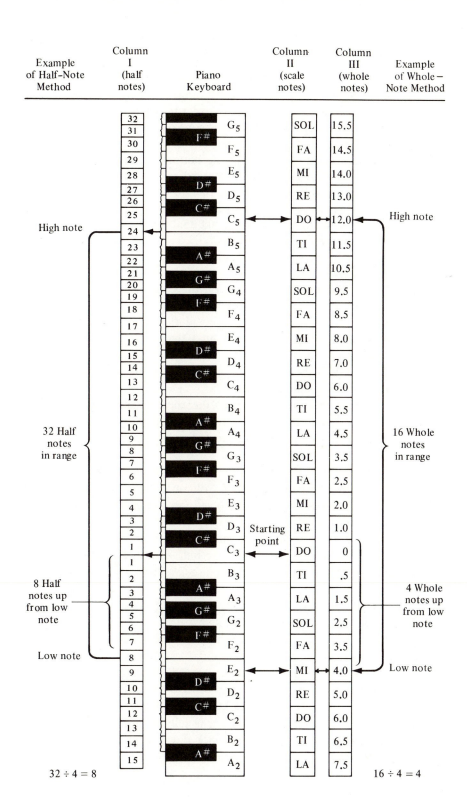

(j) Use this number to determine the number of whole notes to count up from the bottom of the client's range to the optimum pitch level. Use Column III in the chart in order to avoid error in calculating whole note steps on the piano keyboard. Note that *not all* steps on the keyboard are whole notes.

(k) One-fourth the way up from the bottom of the range is the optimum pitch level. The half notes adjacent to this point are also likely to be full and resonant; therefore, the note that is located by Method A and the two half notes flanking it are, theoretically, the best place on the scale for habitual use as a base for inflecting the majority of pitch patterns.

(l) Repeat this process for reliability.

2. Half-note calculation method:

(a) Locate the highest note sung on the chart. Mark the number in Column I corresponding to this note.

(b) Locate the lowest note sung and mark it in Column I.

(c) Take the numbers from Column I that correspond to these two marks and add them.

(d) The result is the total number of half notes in the client's range. Divide this number by 4.

(e) Count *up* from the bottom of the client's range by the number derived in Step d (e.g., by 5, 6, 7, or whatever it is).

(f) The place you locate on the scale by this procedure is the client's optimum pitch.

(g) An example of this procedure is presented in the Optimum Pitch-Location Chart to the *left* of Column I. This method eliminates some of the awkwardness involved in counting by whole notes on a piano keyboard.

3. Some people can sing *ah* better than the notes *do, re, mi,* etc. Follow all steps in either the whole note or half note methods to determine optimum pitch but have the client use *ah* instead of the scale note names.

4. Use numbers in place of *ah* or *do, re, mi* (e.g., *one, two, three,* etc.). These may be spoken on key or sung.

5. Singing steadily up the scale on sustained notes can be very tiring, particularly when trying to negotiate the last three or four notes in the upper part of the range. In order to relieve strain, clinicians often resort to two techniques to ease the process and achieve better results. First, major intervals of a given key are used instead of all the notes in the octave; and second, the teacher usually has the client sing quickly up the scale to the high note and back down again without sustaining any of the notes. This procedure may be outlined as follows:

(a) Locate C₃ (or C₄ for women); have the client hum this note.

(b) Sing the following notes quickly both up and down the scale: C-E-G-C-G-E-C. Keep the voice "light" and do not sustain the high note. Use the vowel, *ah*.

(c) If the client is successful, try C♯ in the same manner, using the intervals, C♯-F-G♯-C♯-G♯-F-C♯. (Note: These are the major intervals of the key of C♯.)[3]

(d) Continue in this manner, moving up one half note each time a key has been completed successfully. When the client is no longer able to "hit" the high note, record the top note of the last scale done satisfactorily. *In order to establish the full range, use falsetto on the highest part of the range.*

(e) Locate the lowest note in the client's pitch range by singing down the scale continuously. It is not necessary to sing major chord intervals in moving *down* the scale because difficulty is at a minimum. Note the last note sung and record.

(f) Use either the whole-note or half-note methods to determine optimum pitch.

6. Optimum pitch may be tentatively located by critical listening.

(a) Have the client block his ear canal on one side by placing his finger tip over the tragus (the projection that partially covers the opening to the canal) and depressing it. An ear plug or ear mold material can also be used to occlude the canal.

(b) Ask him to hum slowly up the scale from the bottom of his range, holding the force of his output constant.

(c) Instruct the client to listen carefully to determine whether there is a level where the intensity swells without increasing effort. Repeat, then locate this note on the piano or by use of a pitch pipe.

(d) The open vowel *ah* can by sung in place of humming while performing Steps a–c.

(e) The clinician may also listen carefully to determine if surging of tone takes place at a given pitch level.

(f) Check the results with the outcomes of other optimum pitch experiments.

---

[3] Major intervals for a full circle of keys is as follows:

Key	Intervals	Key	Intervals
C	C–E–G–C–G–E–C	G	G–B–D–G–D–B–G
C♯	C♯–F–G♯–C♯–G♯–F–C♯	G♯	G♯–C–D♯–G♯–D♯–C–G♯
D	D–F♯–A–D–A–F♯–D	A	A–C♯–E–A–E–C♯–A
D♯	D♯–G–A♯–D♯–A♯–G–D♯	A♯	A♯–D–F–A♯–F–D–A♯
E	E–G♯–B–E–B–G♯–E	B	B–D♯–F♯–B–F♯–D♯–B
F	F–A–C–F–C–A–F	C	C–E–G–C–G–E–C
F♯	F♯–A♯–C♯–F♯–C♯–A♯–F♯		

Interpretation of Optimum Pitch Tests

Ideally, optimum pitch is located at a place in one's range that is the "fullest and richest" when effort is held constant. Voice specialists have found that the optimum level is more than just one finite note and involves at least two or more half notes in the optimum area. If the client's *modal pitch* level is more than two notes from the optimum center (either higher or lower), both clinician and client should consider shifting the modal pitch level to approximate more closely the optimum level. It is also recommended that the client use this level in voice exercises. In shifting to a new modal level, one should test the efficiency, ease, and appropriateness of the new level before insisting upon its use in voice exercises.

Testing Optimum Pitch for Appropriateness

After optimum pitch has been determined by one of the procedures recommended earlier, the clinician and client should then explore the appropriateness, efficiency, and strength of this level.

PROCEDURES

1. Test the strength and efficiency of optimum pitch by the following procedure.
   (a) Locate optimum pitch with a pitch pipe or piano.
   (b) Vocalize an *ah* at a conversational level without attempting to force it.
   (c) Holding force constant, move up the scale one half note at a time (C to C♯, C♯ to D, etc.), at a rate of one note every two seconds. As the client moves away from the optimum pitch level, a perceptible decrease in loudness (also described as fullness and richness) should be observed.
   (d) Repeat Steps a–b; both clinician and client should listen carefully to detect the level at which change occurs.
   (e) In order for the client to hear his voice better, have him stop up one ear by placing his fingertip over the tragus. Repeat Steps a–c and note the results.
2. Optimum pitch may be tested by counting on a monopitch:
   (a) Find optimum pitch.
   (b) Hum on the optimum pitch level in a monotone. Hold the tone steadily on this level without raising or lowering the pitch.
   (c) Hum on optimum pitch in a monotone, then sing the following numbers on that pitch level, *one, two, three, four, five,* slightly prolonging the vowel in each number.
   (d) Count from one to five in a monotone on the optimum pitch level.
   (e) Count in the same manner on the next half note up the scale (C to C♯). Compare the results. Was the voice on one key fuller and richer than the other? Be sure to hold force constant.

(f) If no perceptible difference occurs in Step e, move up the scale another half note (C♯ to D). Compare the results of singing in key C♯ to key D.

(g) Continue to move up the scale one half note at a time until a difference in ease and fullness is detected.

(h) Return to optimum pitch and move down the scale (C to B, etc.) until a change is observed.

(i) Throughout this procedure, the clinician is seeking an answer to the question, "Are the full, resonant tones consistent with the optimum pitch levels as determined by formal tests?"

3. One may also test the efficiency and strength of optimum pitch by using short sentences, samples of which are included at the end of this procedure.

(a) Use the same procedure as given for Procedure 2.

(b) After intoning the sentence on a monopitch, modify pitch by using an inflectional pattern, but keep the steps and glides within a narrow range for control. *Do not change key.*

(c) Perform each sentence with a moderate pitch pattern on a series of half notes (C-C♯-D-D♯-E-F; C-B-A♯-A). Which notes were best in terms of resonance and ease? Do these notes coincide with optimum pitch as determined by formal tests?

(d) Sample sentences:

The mailman usually comes at eight.

I want to go home early tonight.

Where are you going today?

The sun came up at seven fifteen.

It usually rains on Sunday afternoon.

MODAL PITCH

The term modal pitch refers to the general pitch level that one habitually uses while speaking in a majority of life situations. Said differently, modal pitch is the average pitch level one employs to develop the majority of his pitch contours in speech. Variation from this level is normal, but most speakers return to a basic level, usually covering a small range of two or three half notes, to develop the majority of the melody patterns characteristic of their speech.

Ideally, it is desirable to have modal pitch located at the optimum pitch level to facilitate pitch contour development. This placement permits three-fourths of the range for inflecting pitch contours above the base level, yet leaves one-fourth of the range for downglides that usually occur at the ends of phrases and sentences. A study to determine whether or not the modal pitch of a given person is appropriate should be undertaken in conjunction with the effort to locate optimum pitch.

Determining Modal Pitch

Probably the best way to determine modal pitch is to take an adequate sample of the modal speech and determine the average level used in the various sentences employed. Usually, having the client read a nonemotional passage of prose should be sufficient for analysis. However, it is possible that a person might read on one level and converse on another; therefore, it is wise to analyze modal pitch in both modalities.

PROCEDURES FOR DETERMINING MODAL PITCH BY READING

1. Matching modal pitch.
   (a) Have the client read one of the selections on pp. 72–73 and listen carefully to his general pitch level.
   (b) Hum a pitch that seems to approximate his average fundamental frequency level.
   (c) Experiment by raising your level in relation to the client's level. Now, return to the client's level.
   (d) Lower your level in relation to the client's level. Return to his level.
   (e) After several trials of raising and lowering your level in relation to the client's level, prolong the client's level and locate it with a pitch pipe or piano. The result should approximate the client's modal pitch.
2. Averaging key words.
   (a) As the client reads the selection, listen carefully and follow the pitch patterns subvocally by imitating his patterns at a low level of intensity.
   (b) When the client reads one of the words in the selection that seems to characterize his modal pitch level, prolong the vowel of that word and locate the pitch level with the aid of a pitch pipe or piano.
   (c) Repeat Step b several times on selected key words.
   (d) Average out the pitch levels of the total number of samples taken. The result should approximate the modal pitch level of the client.
3. Location of modal pitch with the aid of a tape recorder.
   (a) Make a tape recording of the client as he reads one of the two selections on pp. 72–73.
   (b) Locate the modal pitch level with the aid of a pitch pipe or piano. Since the sample is recorded, make several estimations of the modal pitch level, using either Procedures 1 or 2.

SELECTIONS FOR PRACTICE

1. Have you ever wanted to go where the wild geese go? In autumn when the first traces of frost appear, the geese darken the sky with their

southward flight, their distinctive honk-honk shattering the crisp autumnal air. As you look at the geese and contemplate the lovely winter they will have in the Southern climes while you will be incarcerated in a snow-trapped world, wouldn't you like to fly with the geese?

2. Red Jacket, the Seneca chief, was a very great orator. There are those who have called him the greatest of all Indian orators. He was a shrewd and logical debator and could hold his own not only at the council fire but in the courtroom against any white man, although he could neither read nor write. He was a potent agitator with all the arts of the skilled orator, who ever extolled the might and glory of his nation and fought against white encroachment on the Indian lands.

PROCEDURE FOR DETERMINING
MODAL PITCH BY USING CONVERSATIONAL MATERIALS

Select a topic for conversation—family, sports, ecology, politics—and make a tape recording. Use the same procedures for locating modal pitch as you did in Procedures 1 or 2 above.

The answers to these three questions should be determined: Does modal pitch for reading differ from that used for conversational speech? Does the modal pitch level determined by the analysis fit the modal level used by the client in off-guard speech? Does the modal pitch level coincide with the optimum pitch level derived by formal tests?

PROCEDURE FOR DETERMINING
MODAL PITCH BY THE CHEWING METHOD

The proponents of this method of voice training feel that most persons will spontaneously produce a pitch level that is best for speaking if asked to hum or intone softly while in the process of chewing. The pitch level produced in this very natural activity is often said to coincide with one's optimum pitch or, more simply, with the "best level" for initiating pitch for that person. In order to determine this best-level pitch, try the following procedure:[4]

(a) Have the client chew a piece of gum or a semi-soft piece of candy (licorice, jelly bean).

(b) Be sure he keeps his mouth open, varies his tongue position during the chewing, and uses a reasonable amount of mouth opening.

(c) Continue this activity in order to establish a base line of chewing activity that is natural and free from tension.

(d) Have the client initiate voice as he is chewing, but do not model a tone for him.

(e) Locate the general pitch level with a pitch pipe or piano. The result should approximate "best level" for the client.

[4] For a more detailed procedure of the chewing method, refer to Chapter 11.

If it has been impossible to locate optimum pitch with a given person because of difficulty in handling scale exercises, this procedure can be valuable in indicating a *natural* level that can be used for phonatory exercises.

PITCH CHANGE

The chief means of expressing thought and emotion is through the effective use of various pitch levels and pitch changes. If one continually speaks with little variation in pitch or in a monotone, a loss in communication results. The skillful use of pitch is more effective than other vocal factors, such as quality, rate, or force in conveying a wide range of meaning, subtle nuances of thought, and a variety of emotional states. Failure to use a normal range of pitch variations can lead to monotony and possible vocal abuse through constant repetition.

It is not possible to teach pitch contours per se, because they are closely related to a speaker's thoughts and emotions and should be generated naturally. Training should be aimed at gaining mastery over techniques of manipulating pitch to enhance communication. Care must be taken to avoid using stereotyped patterns or a stilted style of speaking in all forms of oral communication.

Ways of Changing Pitch

There are three ways to change pitch—the step, glide, and altering fundamental frequency. Control over each of these pitch changing approaches must be mastered before the client attempts to develop pitch contours.

The Step

The step is the means whereby a speaker changes pitch by literally stepping from one pitch level to another, without gliding through all the intervening notes. For example, in stepping from C to G, one does not permit his voice to glide through C♯, D, D♯, and E. Step is achieved by diminishing intensity on the first pitch level before stepping to the next level.

EXERCISES

1. Practice changing pitch in steps on the following short phrases:

a. The first one

b. He turned around.

c. The yellow one

d. He doesn't know.

e. A big one

f. Her best friend

g. Mildred's fourth trump

h. The clever boxer

i. A good decision

j. The funny comedian

2. Use step to achieve pitch changes on a series of words within a phrase. The steps may vary according to what the speaker wants to do with them.
   a. The colors of the Star Spangled Banner are red, white and blue.
   b. Thanksgiving day broke, cold, calm, and crisp.
   c. Tom, Jerry, and Hank formed a trio.
   d. And you're hot and you're cross, and you tumble and toss, till there's nothing 'twixt you and the ticking.
   e. And shocking and rocking
      And darting and parting
      And threading and spreading
3. Step may be used to differentiate general pitch levels of phrases within a sentence.
   a. The decorator chose all the colors of the rainbow—pink in Mary's room, lavender in Mom and Pop's, gold in Sadie's, and pale green in mine.
   b. My great Uncle Charlie Jones was a real swinging pioneer, a deadly shot, a wicked poker player, and a pillar of the church.
   c. The formidable chinook, the fighting steelhead, and the colorful sockeye all return to their birthplace to spawn—the mighty Columbia.
   d. Summer is coming, summer is coming.
      I know it, I know it, I know it.
      Light again, leaf again, life again, love again!
   e. Steaming slowly up the Mississippi, the tug rounded the bend, pushed through the deadwood near shore, and docked at Mrs. Snavely's antiquated pier.
   f. The first frost brought our autumnal color change—the quivering aspens turning yellow, the maples a bright red, and the oaks a deep mahogany hue.
   g. Elmer hitched up his pants, stuffed a cardboard box with worms, picked up his pole, and headed for the creek.

The Glide

Glides, or inflections, occur when one changes pitch during the process of phonating. Typically, gliding pitch changes are made on vowels, diphthongs, glides, and nasal consonants. Glides are employed to enhance meaning and emotion. On individual words at the ends of sentences, an upward glide _____✓ usually connotes a question, while a downward glide _____↘ usually indicates completion of thought or a degree of finality. It is possible to use both an upward and downward inflection on the stressed syllable of a word; this is called *circumflex inflection*. These unusual double inflections are often used to express surprise, innuendo, uncertainty, irony, double meaning, and other subtle nuances of feeling or meaning.

EXERCISES

1. Develop control of glides with the following words. The procedure for using this exercise as an operant conditioning sequence is given in Steps a–c.

Frames	Frames	Frames	Frames	Frames
1 now	11 maybe	21 love	31 employ	41 arrested
2 my	12 she	22 found	32 married	42 failure
3 I	13 upward	23 lost	33 gone	43 interpret
4 one	14 ball	24 reach	34 shout	44 astounded
5 any	15 baby	25 home	35 success	45 blemish
6 why	16 you	26 pretty	36 girlfriend	46 criterion
7 how	17 sound	27 funny	37 professor	47 hastily
8 up	18 mine	28 crazy	38 smashed	48 crowded
9 over	19 these	29 balloon	39 loveliness	49 surprise
10 time	20 please	30 woman	40 harried	50 emphasis

(a) Try the first ten frames with a downward glide. Be sure to diminish the loudness of the tone as the client glides downward. Try to finish the glide before glottal fry occurs (usually on the lowest note in the client's range). Try the next ten frames with an even greater downward glide; continue working in blocks of ten until the client has achieved ease and control in handling glides of at least one octave in magnitude.

(b) Continue working in blocks of ten frames, only this time use an upward inflection; increase the glide range with the next ten frames. Be sure to diminish the loudness of the tone in gliding up; the tone may be diminished to a falsetto. Continue working until maximum upward glides are achieved—strive for at least one octave.

(c) Perform the words in blocks of ten using a circumflex inflection. You may wish to practice circumflex first on a vowel before attempting the words in order to gain control of reversing the glide. When performing disyllabic or polysyllabic words, more control is needed to glide in an appropriate manner. The clinician may elect to model the more difficult words.

2. After mastering control of glides, make up sentences with each of the words contained in Exercise 1. Try the sentence three ways, first with a rising inflection, then with a falling inflection, and finally with a circumflex inflection. Examples:

a. She said yes. She said yes. She said yes.

b. He's wealthy. He's wealthy. He's wealthy.

c. John is honest. John is honest. John is honest.

3. Use glides on the italicized words in the following sentences:
    a. The *funny* clown *leapt* atop the lion's cage.
    b. The *balloon* broke loose, *carrying* Richard in the gondola.
    c. *Why? Why* did he *go?*
    d. *Surprised*, you say? I've *never* been so *surprised* in my life!
    e. *How beautiful* she seemed that night!

Changing Fundamental Frequency

The modal pitch level used by the speaker serves as the base for the majority of his inflectional patterns. Any segment of speech can be shifted from one level to another without changing the intervals of the pitch contour.

EXERCISES

1. Hum C_3 (or C_4 for women) on a monopitch. Chant the sentence below on a monopitch. Without changing key, develop a pitch contour as follows:

    Where are you going?

    Now repeat this pitch contour at the next key up, $C\sharp$, without changing the intervals. If you have been successful in maintaining intervals, you have shifted the modal level from C to $C\sharp$. Try the sentence on D, then $D\sharp$, keeping pitch contours intact. Continue experimenting with other pitch levels but do not change the basic pitch contour.

2. Perform the following sentences on several pitch levels attempting to hold the pitch contour evolved on the first key the same as on the other pitch levels.
    a. The church bell tolled at 11 o'clock.
    b. The school's colors were red and white.
    c. She lifted her eyes to the horizon beyond.
    d. The corn stalks turned brown late in August.
    e. You can find out from Charlie.

3. Read each of the following paragraphs on *one* basic pitch level, in-

flecting a basic pitch contour. Now, try to shift the same paragraph to different keys without changing contours.

a. Oh, how I had looked forward to that 4th of July picnic! All the old gang promised to come—Joe, Ellen, Harry, Meg—even Tom from three hundred miles away. Weather permitting was the only condition! July 4th broke in a rain-bedecked sky. Thunder clapped and lightning of all varieties sizzled across the heavens. And then torrents of rain! Hurricane warnings were posted. Then I knew our reunion would have to wait another year—to the next 4th of July. Disappointed? What do you think?

b. It was spring and the whole world was brimming with life. The rainswept skies with their departing thunderheads were turning a cobalt blue. Gentle breezes were rustling the lacy pink and white dogwoods in the forest, and the cardinal sat on the old oak's highest branch whistling to his mate. The fragrance of crabapple and plum blossoms permeated the moisture-laden air. It was the best of all seasons, and it was fun just being alive.

c. The lovely redbud tree with its clusters of rose-purple flowers that seem to grow right out of the dark bark of the branches is a spring delight to many sections of the more temperate areas of our country. In reading about this spectacular tree, I was amazed to find its sad legend—that of the Judas tree. The Judas tree grew in the Middle East, and it was from this tree that Judas hanged himself, and its then white flowers turned color with shame and have blushed ever since. And that is why the redbud is the color that it is.

INTONATION

The term intonation embraces the entire range of pitch inflections used by a speaker. It is concerned with changes in pitch and the contours that evolve from these changes from one phrase to another. Before beginning pitch contour exercises, several basic principles should be studied:

1. Intonation of phrases occurs at three general pitch levels, low, middle, and high. It is possible to generate a fourth general level, very high, which is associated with unusual or extreme conditions, such as great surprise or shock.

2. When utilizing a general pitch level, a speaker will initiate a contour at a pitch level known as a pitch point.

3. A contour, also called a clause or phrase, always contains at least two pitch points.

4. Contours are terminated by pauses or transitions.

5. Transitions may be made with rising, falling, or sustained (unchanging) pitch inflections. Even the smallest contour has at least two pitch levels and one terminal.

EXERCISES ON THE USE OF RISING INFLECTIONS

1. Rising inflections are often used to indicate a question:

a. Did she arrive?

b. Did you find it?

c. Is there any more?

d. Do you dance?

e. Where is my coat?

f. Have you lost it?

g. Doesn't he live there?

h. Why not now?

i. Do you think they will come tomorrow?

j. John won't go?

2. Rising inflections are often used to terminate a contour:

a. Do you think she will come tomorrow?

b. Did you say that clearly?

c. How do you know?

d. When will he come?

e. What do you think will happen?

3. Rising inflections are used to achieve a higher pitch level in anticipation of stress within contours:

a. My blue sweater

b. I seldom go.

c. Mazie grinned sheepishly.

d. You smoothie, you

e. The only honest judge

f. A snarling vicious dog

g. The old wrinkled man

h. A long, long time ago

i. Ruby laughed and laughed.

j. of a beautiful and serene morning

4. Rising inflections are often directly related to stress:

a. The first prize

b. The red, yellow, and blue

c. The pretty dress

d. My oldest and dearest friend

e. I love doughnuts.

f. She kissed him.

EXERCISES ON THE USE OF FALLING INFLECTIONS

1. Falling inflections are used to indicate finality or positive statement:

a. I don't think so.

b. It's the best one.

c. Compared to Ford

d. Come over here.

e. I think it's beautiful.

f. He's not the smartest one.

g. He grew angry.

h. I like chocolate pie.

i. Don't touch it.

j. You must be starved.

2. Falling inflections are often used to terminate phrases:

a. in the fall

b. on the man

c. on Main Street

d. the difficult exam

e. the poor soul

f. of the day

g. in the barnyard

h. of the players

i. came to a stop

j. by crumbling walls

3. By increasing falling inflections, greater stress can be achieved:

a. No!

b. Yes!

c. How!

d. Never!

e. Married!

f. Positively not!

g. I'll never go!

h. It's a shocking situation!

i. The sign says "Stop!"

j. But the barn was blue!

4. Falling inflections are used to move from a high general level to a lower one within a phrase:

a. The | orange, yellow, | and | red ↘

b. John! Mark! Bill! | Come | here. ↘

c. It's | almost impossible to | do | it. ↘

d. Never | in the | history | of | man ↘

e. The | paratrooper | twisted | and | turned | as he fell. ↘

EXERCISES ON SUSTAINED PITCH

1. Sustained pitch is used to convey indecision (terminal use):

a. You   might be right . . . . ⟶

b. I thought I knew . . . . ⟶

c. On the other hand, we could come . . . . ⟶

d. Oh, give me the red one, or the blue . . . . ⟶

e. I might have two dollars, maybe more . . . . ⟶

2. Sustained pitch can be used to indicate unfinished thought (terminal use):

a. He said that ⟶   f. Mecham didn't ⟶

b. Well, er, that is ⟶   g. I wonder if you'd ⟶

c. It was about, er ⟶   h. Not that Jack could ⟶

d. James ought ⟶   i. Oh, I didn't know it was ⟶

e. As I was saying, I ⟶   j. Two or three days, maybe ⟶

3. Sustained pitch often precedes stressed elements in phrases:

a. It was a | fine day.   c. when the | clouds

b. if you could | only   d. out of | nowhere

e. in a↑blue   h. from a↑great man

f. of a↑good day   i. not what↑I think

g. to a↑friend   j. of the↑ten men

4. Sustained pitch can often be used to implement strong stress:

a. Don't you dare do it! ⟶

b. I cry unto you! ⟶

c. Come here this minute! ⟶

d. You sniveling liar! ⟶

Use of General Pitch Levels

A speaker may change the general pitch level of his voice for a number of reasons. On the other hand, a speaker may choose to remain on one level for·entirely different reasons. The four levels traditionally recognized by linguists—low, middle, high, and very high—relate to general levels of the total pitch range of the individual.[5] Practice the material contained in each of the following exercises on general pitch level usage.

EXERCISES

1. Pitch changes that convey meaning or emotion generally utilize more than one general pitch level:

a. The | first one ↘

b. He | cried a|loud. ↘

c. Come | over here! ↘

d. The | play | was a | huge | success. ↘

e. I | trem|ble at the | sight | of him. ↘

2. Pitch can be sustained on one level, provided the steps or glides are small or limited:

Oh, I don't know. ↘

[5] General pitch level as used in this context refers to low, middle, and upper ranges of the speaking voice. The very high level refers to an upper part of the range that is used for special or unusual purposes.

3. General pitch changes are often used to show contrast:

   a. For richer or poorer

   b. The winners and the losers

   c. The red, orange, and gold of fall

   d. Nickels, dimes, quarters, and half dollars

   e. Large, medium, and small sizes

4. The use of stress usually calls for a change in general pitch level:

   a. Bart shouted, "William, come back here!"

   b. He paused noticeably, then vaulted over the fence.

   c. "Be sure to call the office," she cried as he departed.

   d. If you think I'm going, you're crazy.

   e. "Go back! Go back!" the base coach yelled.

5. Emotional content will often influence the selection of a general pitch level:

   a. Oh that this too, too solid flesh would melt!

   b. Tomorrow, and tomorrow, and tomorrow—

   c. Richie, the Giants lost last night.

   d. Marvelous! Stupendous! Unbelievable!

   e. Oh! That's funny! Hilarious!

6. Expansion of a sentence is often accompanied by a general pitch level change on the expanded portion to facilitate meaning:

   a. I accept your answer.

      I accept your answer, but I'll never believe it.

b. First, you put in milk.

First, you put in milk, then add the cheese later.

c. One minute you say she's here.

One minute you say she's here, then the next

minute you say she's gone.

d. She has a peaches and cream complexion.

She has a peaches and cream complexion, and the

most beautiful eyes I have ever seen.

e. George went to Ondine's and ordered.

George went to Ondine's and ordered a Crab Louis

and a bottle of California's finest Grey Riesling.

Inflection and Emotion

While pitch changes are utilized freely and consciously by most speakers to bring out meaning, various emotional states can have a profound effect upon an individual and consequently can have much to do with the pitch contours he generates. Since we all do not react the same way to given situations, a wide variety of responses is possible.

EXERCISES

1. In each of the sentences below, attempt to capture the emotional states suggested by the following words:

anger	fear	irony	sadness
bitterness	frustration	joy	surprise
envy	hostility	love	shock

   a. You know what it means.
   b. Many of them have gone.
   c. I could have laughed.
   d. The administrator made the right decision.
   e. What do you make of that?
   f. How do you do?
   g. I'll think it over.
   h. Is there any question?

i.   What do you mean by that?

j.   Are you going to go?

2. The following short selections involve a range of emotions. Read over each selection silently to capture the emotion intended by each author, then give yourself over to the reading of it.

a. In Reading gaol by Reading town
    There is a pit of shame,
And in it lies a wretched man
    Eaten by teeth of flame,
In a burning winding-sheet he lies,
    And his grave has got no name.

And there, till Christ call forth the dead,
    In silence let him lie.
No need to waste the foolish tear,
    Or heave a windy sigh;
The man had killed the thing he loved,
    And so he had to die.

And all men kill the thing they love,
    By all let this be heard,
Some do it with a bitter look,
    Some with a flattering word,
The coward does it with a kiss,
    The brave man with a sword!
        —from Oscar Wilde, "The Ballad of Reading Gaol"

b. Water, water, everywhere,
And all the boards did
       shrink;
Water, water, everywhere,
Nor any drop to drink.

The very deep did rot: O Christ!
That ever this should be!
Yea, slimy things did crawl with legs
Upon the slimy sea.
      —from Samuel Taylor Coleridge, "Rime of
      the Ancient Mariner"

c. The sea! the sea! the open sea!
The blue, the fresh, the ever free!
Without a mark, without a bound,
It runneth the earth's wide regions round;
It plays with the clouds; it mocks the skies;
Or like a cradled creature lies.

I'm on the sea! I'm on the sea!
I am where I would ever be;
With the blue above and the blue below,
And silence wheresoe'er I go;
If a storm should come and awake the deep,
What matter? I shall ride and sleep.

I love, O how I love to ride
On the fierce, foaming, bursting tide,
When every mad wave drowns the moon
Or whistles aloft his tempest tune,
And tells how goeth the world below,
And why the sou'west blasts do blow.
        —Bryan Waller Proctor, "The Sea"

Faulty Pitch Patterns

The most obvious pitch fault is vocal monotony due to consistent lack of pitch variation. Speaking on one pitch level without inflection is the most extreme form of this problem and is occasionally encountered in the person with the hoarse voice. Not only does the person with a monotonous voice lull his auditors to sleep, he invariably adds to his voice problem by the strain attendant with the use of only one pitch. Variety can relieve voice strain due to monotony and will do much to heighten the meaning and emotional content of what the speaker has to say.

EXERCISES

1. Read the selections below under the following conditions: (a) use extreme monotony (try to speak on a monopitch); (b) use a narrow pitch range and a modicum of pitch-pattern variation; and (c) use a broad pitch range and attempt to increase pitch variation. Avoid a stilted performance. The clinician should make a tape recording and play back the results for analysis and comments.

   a. A foolish consistency is the hobgoblin of little minds, adored by little statesmen and philosophers and divines. With consistency a great soul has simply nothing to do. He may as well concern himself with his shadow on the wall. Speak what you think now in hard words and to-morrow speak what to-morrow thinks in hard words again, though it contradict every thing you said to-day.—'Ah, so you shall be sure to be misunderstood.'—Is it so bad then to be misunderstood? Pythagoras was misunderstood, and Socrates, and Jesus, and Luther, and Copernicus, and Galileo, and Newton, and every pure and wise spirit that ever took flesh. To be great is to be misunderstood.
        —from Ralph Waldo Emerson, "Self-Reliance"

b.   To every thing there is a season, and a time to every purpose
under the heaven:
A time to be born, and a time to die; a time to plant, and a
time to pluck that which is planted;
A time to kill, and a time to heal; a time to break down, and
a time to build up;
A time to weep, and a time to laugh; a time to mourn, and a
time to dance;
A time to cast away stones, and a time to gather stones together;
a time to embrace, and a time to refrain from embracing;
A time to get, and a time to lose; a time to keep, and a time
to throw away;
A time to rend, and a time to sew; a time to keep silence, and
a time to speak;
A time to love, and a time to hate; a time of war, and a time
of peace.
        —from Ecclesiastes, the Bible

c.   Gaily bedight,
      A gallant knight,
In sunshine and in shadow,
      Had journeyed long,
      Singing a song,
In search of Eldorado.

      But he grew old—
      This knight so bold—
And o'er his heart a shadow
      Fell as he found
      No spot of ground
That looked like Eldorado.

      And, as his strength
      Failed him at length,
He met a pilgrim shadow—
      "Shadow," said he,
      "Where can it be—
This land of Eldorado?"

      "Over the Mountains
      Of the Moon,
Down the Valley of the Shadow,
      Ride, boldly ride,"
      The shade replied—
"If you seek for Eldorado."
        —Edgar Allan Poe, "Eldorado"

2. The overuse of indefinite glides or sustained pitch in terminal positions of phrases or sentences containing statements suggests lack of conviction or uncertainty on the part of the speaker and is to be avoided. Use a sustained pitch level on the final words on the internal phrases and at the ends of the sentences below. Make a tape recording and analyze the results. Perform the sentences a second time using positive downglides. Analyze the results. Which seemed to carry the most conviction? Which was the more interesting?

   a. The fog usually comes in at four o'clock in the morning, but doesn't stay too long, usually burning off by 10 o'clock.
   b. I want you to get several things at the store—a bunch of carrots, French green beans, a head of lettuce, and a small bag of potatoes.
   c. I love a band—a brass band. I love to hear it play when I go to the park on Sunday mornings. I could listen to it all day.
   d. It was many and many a year ago,
        In a kingdom by the sea,
      That a maid there lived whom you may know
        By the name of Annabel Lee.
   e. The fisherman cast his net into the sea, hoping for a generous catch; the surf was rough, the fishing tough, but perseverance won the day.

3. Failure to vary step or glide can lead to vocal monotony and ineffective speech. This fault usually occurs when the speaker uses the same interval in changing from one general level to the other (usually in going from a middle to a high general level). In order to break up the monotony of a repetitious interval, practice variation of interval in the following short phrases and sentences:

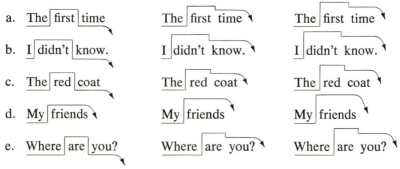

4. Mark the words that you want to stress in the two prose selections that are included in Exercise 5 that follows. Then attempt to vary the intervals in the pitch contours. Try varying the intervals in more than one way.

5. The use of too high or too low modal level can lead to several problems

in pitch management. If the modal level is placed too high, difficulty and, possibly, vocal strain will accompany attempts to inflect upward in order to bring out meaning. The use of a modal pitch level that is too low can lead to (a) vocal strain and discomfort, (b) ineffective downglides in declarative statements (because there is insufficient lower range), and (c) pitch breaks or glottal fry on downglides when the lowest note in the range is reached. Read the selections below in two ways: (a) Read each selection two or three notes below your modal level; (b) read each selection at a modal level bordering the high part of your range. Observe how the ability to handle pitch contours in a normal or interesting fashion is greatly decreased.

a. The coast highway north from Gold Beach is unforgettably beautiful, winding its way along the rugged seacoast through lush forests of fir, darting inland for a few miles past sparkling mountain lakes, then wending its way back again to the turbulent sea pounding the long strips of hard-packed sand. What a sense of freedom and adventure we had as we rolled north, for each mile brought a new experience in pictorial beauty. We stopped many times to take deep breaths of crisp, fresh air, or to vigorously hike a few hundred yards along the beach.

b. Two of our most spectacular National Parks are Sequoia and Kings, running from the gentle foothills of the San Joaquin Valley to the splintered crest of the Sierra Nevada in California. They adjoin and are often referred to as twin parks. Both of the parks are noted for lakes, waterfalls and rushing rivers, canyons, and giant trees. Sequoia's name comes from the Sequoia Gigantea, close relative to the redwood. These are massive trees; some are higher than a twenty-story building. Largest of these giantics is the General Sherman Tree, over thirty-six feet through and one hundred and one feet around at the base. It is not only the size of these trees that astonish the visitor, but their age as well. General Sherman tree started its upward thrust to the skies when the Trojans and Greeks were battling. How humble one feels in his presence!

RATE

Rate of utterance is concerned with the duration or time element of any given segment of speech and is easily quantified by measurement. Voice clinicians should be concerned with the entire range of rates, from the smallest element of speech, the phoneme, to the longest, an entire oral presentation. In working with rate we are concerned with the duration of syllables, words, phrases, and sentences, as well as with overall rates used and speaking. Choice of rate should be directly related to both and emotion. Speech rates may be analyzed in terms of milli-seconds, seconds, minutes, and even hours.

Voice Problems Associated with Rate

Voice problems associated with rate occur along a continuum of analysis from the one extreme of "too fast" to the other of "too slow." Generally, problems lie in the direction of the "too fast" end of the continuum. Speed of utterance is directly related to content, the listener, and the situation; therefore, a variety of rates is possible and desirable in communication.

Probably the most important area of concern for the voice clinician is the duration of the syllable. Syllable length, for example, can be appreciably changed by durational stress, which in turn increases time of utterance of the word and reduces overall word rate in speaking. The clinician should avoid telling the client to "slow down"—he must show him how to do so. The client needs to know the differences in time between stressed and unstressed syllables.

Rate Control

A speaker's rate should be determined by his thoughts and emotions rather than by deliberately manipulating the voice mechanically. In order to gain insight into the factors governing rate, perform Exercises 1–8. The materials in Chapter 10 should also prove especially helpful in achieving greater rate control, especially the sections on phonetic power, pp. 185–186, developing oral and pharyngeal resonance, pp. 167–169, and duration and sustained resonance, pp. 169–171.

EXERCISES

1. Study the duration of vowels and consonants in relation to each other. Model the words below for the client, utilizing good duration for the more sonorous sounds. Have the client echo the response as closely as possible. Contrast the short vowels with the long ones. Which consonants have the greatest duration? The least? In performing these words, have the client experiment with more than one duration of the phonemic elements in the words in order to develop greater awareness and control of rate.

Frames	Frames	Frames	Frames	Frames
1 sit	5 let	9 could	13 at	17 thin
2 meat	6 tomb	10 champ	14 cat	18 coot
3 mean	7 map	11 say	15 think	19 sear
4 tame	8 shape	12 dope	16 though	20 my

21 long	27 wear	33 mink	39 myth	45 file
22 paw	28 shout	34 morn	40 pout	46 tap
23 laugh	29 dike	35 suit	41 putt	47 oust
24 tip	30 who	36 mouth	42 guest	48 feud
25 tote	31 sport	37 gale	43 least	49 dial
26 din	32 law	38 lip	44 get	50 mice

2. The stressed syllables in disyllabic and polysyllabic words are invariably longer in duration than the unstressed syllables. Have the client perform the following words, giving greater duration to stressed syllables. Speed up syllable rate of the unstressed syllables.

Frames	Frames	Frames	Frames	Frames
1 harmony	11 morning	21 gallon	31 dapper	41 ripple
2 simple	12 federal	22 limpid	32 celestial	42 dreary
3 daring	13 murmur	23 cancel	33 fragmental	43 infinite
4 infer	14 syphon	24 mystical	34 complication	44 heavenly
5 courage	15 fluent	25 finite	35 abound	45 hormone
6 delight	16 balloon	26 raindrop	36 understand	46 material
7 flourish	17 thimble	27 alone	37 concur	47 accent
8 happy	18 carousel	28 bountiful	38 bastion	48 acoustical
9 spirit	19 monsoon	29 calling	39 bombast	49 pantry
10 convention	20 bulwark	30 symphony	40 plunder	50 padlock

3. There is a direct relationship between phrase rate and meaning. Usually, phrases that contain little meaning are spoken at a faster rate than those that are more meaningful. The following sentences contain many "filler" phrases that are typically employed by most speakers, such as *meanwhile, moreover, nevertheless, as I said before.* Have the client read the following sentences, saying the filler phrases more quickly than the meaningful material.

a. By the way, who won the Tournament of Champions this year?

b. After all is said and done, who cares about the why's and wherefore's?

c. As I mentioned before, Ralph balked, which was nothing new, and walked the winning run home.

d. If one were to ponder the situation and to think more seriously about values, he would recognize, I am sure, the grandeur and sublimity of—and I am sure you will agree with me—abstract art.

e. In the meantime, while you were treading water, Gary won the race.

f. The venerable professor, she noted, talked about antiquity with a reverence that was noticeably absent when he spoke about modernity.

g. Interestingly enough, the salvage crew did find the Spanish galleon and all the gold, too.

h. Ruby turned, as was her wont, dropped her handkerchief, the little flirt, giggled noticeably, and walked mincingly on.

i. As I said before, and you weren't listening, high tide is at nine o'clock.

j. Well, we must think it over, I think, and really think it through.

4. Not all phrases in sentences are equally important or meaningful. Study the following sentences with the client, underlining the most meaningful phrases. Then have the client read the sentences aloud, attempting to give greater duration to the more meaningful phrases.

a. Potatoes, asparagus, cabbage, green peppers, lettuce—you name it—all vegetables are sky-high compared to three years ago.

b. The site of the raid was down along the riverside, close to the dark mass of factory buildings; it was a squalid rooming house crammed with newly arrived foreigners who often slept three or four to a room in spite of police regulations.

c. All appeared to be most serene, then a loud clap of thunder and jagged streaks of lightning brought all to their feet.

d. Stand up and be counted, or take the coward's way out and remain seated.

e. Charles thought quietly for a moment, then suddenly leapt to his feet.

f. And now abideth faith, hope, charity, these three; but the greatest of these is charity.

g. You can use red, blue, or gold—any bright color—but the fact remains that the touches of crystal themselves are the most dominant accents in the room.

h. Masterson picked up the objects, one by one, with the greatest care, slipped each of them into a brown paper bag, and put it into his briefcase.

i. You may talk all you want about Williams, Rubin, or Steinberg, but you have never heard anyone play the violin until you have heard Adolph Moorehead.

5. The emotional content of spoken material can greatly influence rate. Usually, the "heavier" emotions, such as grief, sadness, or solemnity, are associated with slower rates, while the "lighter" emotions, such as happiness, gaiety, excitement, and the like, are associated with faster rates. Have the client attempt to vary rate to suit the emotional content, as it appears to him, on the following sentences:

a. She darted across the street quickly, turned furtively, caught a glimpse of her pursuer, then ran frantically down the narrow alley, only to find a dead end.

b. The dancers whirled and beat their feet rhythmically to the ever increasing tempo of the music.

c. It was without a doubt, the funniest farce I've ever seen!

d. Jack! Jill! Come here and see the kittens playing with Grandma's yarn.

e. Lucy, guess what? Grandma's going to make homemade strawberry ice cream for your birthday party!

f. Bramson opened the letter, knowing that it contained bad news.

g. The procession rounded the turn and came up the aisle, with the lesser dignitaries preceding the President and his distinguished guests.

h. Marcia sobbed for hours over the loss of her favorite rag doll.

i. The sombre tones of the Requiem Mass reverberated throughout the cathedral, leaving all solemn, sad, and bereft.

j. With leaden feet, the vanquished trudged that last long mile of retreat.

6. Oral reading rate for nonemotional, factual material averages approximately 165 words per minute, with a range of 150 to 180 wpm. In order to be effective, rates slower than 150 require greater stress and judicious use of pause to keep the reading from seeming too slow. Rates in excess of 180 wpm require even greater skill in order to permit the listeners to follow the meaning. Have the client read aloud one of the selections below. Instruct the client to read at his usual oral reading rate in a conversational voice. Signal the client when to begin in order to time the number of words read in sixty seconds, using a stopwatch or a wrist watch with a sweep second hand. Mark the last word read at the sixty-second interval, then count the total number of words read. The result is the oral reading rate. The experiment should be tried at least twice. If the results do not fall within the 150-180 wpm range, work on reading rate until the client can read with normal range.

a. The condition of our physical environment is reflected in the condition of man; if the physical environment is healthy, man likely will be healthy. Thus we must look to the future and become more aware of the unity of human needs. The erosion of fields, forests, and mountains and the pollution of our air, streams, lakes, and oceans work as a chain reaction throughout our nation and the world. Pollution knows no geographic nor national boundaries. It is no respector of person. We cannot isolate ourselves from this gigantic problem for it involves all mankind. The smoke of one major city can pollute the environment of another—even moving into an adjacent country. The pollution of one of our major rivers dumping into the Gulf of California may kill shrimp, which the Mexicans have depended upon as part of their livelihood. And thus it goes on and on! What will be the outcome, nobody knows. One thing is certain, this is a problem involving one and all. We must monitor all our actions; use less gasoline and gasoline of a lower octane rating; recycle our bottles; not only refrain from littering, but pick up litter that we see; do not throw trash away or burn it; do not throw objects into our waterways—these are just a few of the things we can do to monitor our own actions, which will aid in eliminating this evil.

b. He was a very silent man by custom. All day he hung round the cove, or upon the cliffs, with a brass telescope; all evening he sat in a corner of the parlor next to the fire, and drank rum and water very strong. Mostly he would not speak when spoken to; only look up sudden and fierce, and blow through his nose like a fog horn; and we and the people who came about our house soon learned to let him be. Every day, when he came back from his stroll, he would ask if any seafaring men had gone by along the road. At first we thought it was the want of company of his own kind that made him ask this question; but at last we began to see he was desirous to avoid them. When a seaman put up at the "Admiral Benbow" (as now and then some did, making by the coast road from Bristol), he would look in at him through the curtained door before he entered the parlor; and he was always sure to be as silent as a mouse when any such was present. For me, at least, there was no secret about the matter; for I was, in a way, a sharer in his alarms. He had taken me aside one day, and promised me a silver fourpenny on the first of every month if I would only keep my "weather-eye open for a seafaring man with one leg," and let him know the moment he appeared. Often enough, when the first of the month came round, and I applied to him for my wage, he would only blow through his nose at me, and stare me down; but before the week was out he was sure to think better of it, bring me my fourpenny piece, and repeat his orders to look out for "the seafaring man with one leg."
—from Robert Louis Stevenson, *Treasure Island*

7. Oral reading rate is greatly influenced by content, as the more complex, subtle, or deep the meaning, the more the rate tends to be decreased. Less meaningful materials can be presented at relatively faster rates. The two selections below differ in content. Time each one and compare the results. If both are read at the same rate, have the client work on meaning, particularly through durational stress. After a practice period, time the two selections again and compare the results.

a. The principal contribution that meat makes to health is the protein of lean meats. The human body is built of protein supplied by foods. The health of the muscles, internal organs, hair, nails, blood cells, antibodies, and hormones (each is made of protein) is limited by the kind and amount of protein eaten. An extensive survey made by the United States Department of Agriculture indicates that nine out of every ten Americans suffer from protein deficiencies. Proteins are not harmed when meats are cooked at low temperatures; at high temperatures some of the essential amino acids are broken apart by heat, and their health-promoting value is decreased. Overcooking can also harm the proteins. Try not to cook any meat longer than is necessary to make it tender. With the exception of pork, meats served rare are nutritionally superior to well-done meats. Meat is a rich source of the B vitamins. Most of the B vitamins are not harmed even by long cooking at low temperature except at the surface of the meat. Above the boiling point, the destruction of several B vitamins increases in proportion to the temperature.

b. You have taken me prisoner, with all my warriors. I am much grieved; for I expected, if I did not defeat you, to hold out much longer, and give you more trouble, before I surrendered. I tried hard to bring you into ambush, but your last general understood Indian fighting. I determined to rush on you, and fight you face to face. I fought hard. But your guns were well aimed. The bullets flew like birds in the air, and whizzed by our ears like the wind through the trees in winter. My warriors fell around me; it began to look dismal.

I saw my evil day at hand. The sun rose dim on us in the morning, and at night it sank in a dark cloud, and looked like a ball of fire. That was the last sun that shone on Black Hawk. His heart is dead, and no longer beats quick in his bosom. He is now a prisoner of the white men; they will do with him as they wish. But he can stand torture, and is not afraid of death. He is no coward. Black Hawk is an Indian. He has done nothing for which an Indian ought to be ashamed. He has fought for his countrymen, against white men, who came, year after year, to cheat them and take away their lands. . . .

The spirits of our fathers arose, and spoke to us to avenge our wrongs or die. We set up the war-whoop, and dug up the tomahawk; our knives were ready and the heart of Black Hawk swelled high in his bosom, when he led his warriors to battle. He is satisfied. He will go to the world of spirits contended. He has done his duty. His father will meet him there and commend him.

Black Hawk is a true Indian, and disdains to cry like a woman. He feels for his wife, his children, and his friends. But he does not care for himself. He cares for the Nation and the Indians. They will suffer. He laments their fate. Farewell, my Nation! Black Hawk tried to save you, and avenge your wrongs. He drank the blood of some of the whites. He has been taken prisoner, and his plans are crushed. He can do no more. He is near his end. His sun is setting and he will rise no more. Farewell to Black Hawk.

—from Black Hawk, "Black Hawk Surrenders"

8. Oral speaking rates vary more than oral reading rates, chiefly because the speaker is involved with generating sentences to express his ideas. The average number of words of speakers on nonemotional, factual material ranges from 140 to 160 words per minute. Have the client choose a topic (e.g., politics, people, vacation), jot down a few ideas, and arrange them in sequence. Make a tape recording of an actual performance (i.e., the monologue delivered to the clinician). Give the client a signal to start and record the words spoken at 60 seconds, 120 seconds, and 180 seconds. On replay, tally the number of words for each one-minute segment. Average the three figures into one. The result is an approximation of the client's speaking rate. If the rate is well below 140 wpm or above 160 wpm, the causes should be studied to prepare for additional work.

FORCE

The term force is used for various aspects of the physical term intensity or the psychological term loudness. The words *amplitude* and *volume* may also be used to convey much the same meaning, but will not be used in this chapter because of the confusion that might arise. The client with a voice disorder who suffers vocal strain or discomfort can do much to alleviate his condition through the judicious use of force. Indeed, because of the pressures of communication, this type of client must learn to use force effectively in order to handle the range of everyday speaking situations successfully as well as the more difficult or trying ones.

Voice Problems Associated with Force

There are several problems associated with force: (a) too loud, (b) too soft, and (c) inability to use force effectively. Injudicious use of voice includes speaking at too high an intensity level to suit the situation, using too much intensity stress, and failing to vary intensity levels. On the other hand there are clients who are not able to use sufficient force to suit the occasion.[6] Finally, there are many individuals who do not know how to use

---

[6] See also Chapter 1 for a discussion of laryngeal valving, and subglottic air pressure and force.

force effectively (e.g., to shade meaning to achieve emphasis or to project voice).

Vocal force may be used in various ways to make speech more effective. The most common use of force by normal speakers is in the stressing of key words, or syllables in words, to bring out meaning or to emphasize a point. Emphasis through force may be extended to important phrases or sentences, or even to an entire section of a speech, particularly the climax portion. Speakers must also learn to use force appropriately, for size of audience and speaking situations vary sufficiently to require adjustment to the conditions at hand.

The Use of Force

Syllable Stress

Most disyllabic and polysyllabic words require force on a given syllable or syllables within the word. By carefully selecting the appropriate syllable to be stressed, one may not only shade meaning better, but may also relieve vocal strain by decreasing vocal power on unstressed syllables. Force, pitch, and duration are usually interrelated in stressing syllables.

EXERCISE

Study the words in the two- to five-syllable frames, underlining the syllables to be stressed. Perform each word, attempting to increase the difference in force between stressed and unstressed syllables. After developing skill, try the words in short phrases or sentences, attempting to maintain the same production as was obtained on individual word production.

Two-syllable frames	Three-syllable frames	Four-syllable frames	Five-syllable frames
1 beauty	1 harmony	1 introduction	1 insinuation
2 person	2 sympathy	2 criterion	2 insignificant
3 color	3 celestial	3 intensity	3 governmentalize
4 perfect	4 redeeming	4 vernacular	4 inseparable
5 tremble	5 production	5 festivity	5 manifestation
6 faulty	6 attempting	6 hypertension	6 neurological
7 reserve	7 crocodile	7 insidious	7 participation
8 spirit	8 crinoline	8 laudatory	8 indestructible
9 daring	9 gyration	9 participle	9 probability
10 imbue	10 interim	10 stupendously	10 repository
11 building	11 nomadic	11 intuitive	11 repudiation
12 shingle	12 potentate	12 territory	12 transfiguration
13 gable	13 tomahawk	13 tolerable	13 fundamentally
14 obtain	14 verbalize	14 preparation	14 laboratory

Two-syllable frames	Three-syllable frames	Four-syllable frames	Five-syllable frames
15 level	15 eccentric	15 innocuous	15 objectivity
16 substance	16 molecule	16 insanity	16 specification
17 callous	17 stimulus	17 insensible	17 distinguishable
18 crinkle	18 sycamore	18 gelatinous	18 pyromaniac
19 decrease	19 lateral	19 historical	19 discrimination
20 prolong	20 otherwise	20 manipulate	20 generosity

Word Stress

The client who tires easily or suffers quality deterioration through prolonged use of voice may be taught to rely upon stress to alleviate some of the "wear and tear" of everyday talking. This may be done by reducing the overall force level somewhat on the less important words in the sentence and relying more upon stressing the important words.

EXERCISE

Perform the following sentences in two ways, first with uniform emphasis and moderate use of force; then with selective meaningful emphasis on key words[7] with less overall force.

a. She didn't say she would go; she said that she might.
b. I don't accept his version of the accident, for I saw it.
c. Don't go too close to the edge.
d. Teddy looked longingly at the double ice cream cone that Bessie was eating.
e. The waves rolled across the glistening sand with ever-increasing force.
f. Just what do you hope to gain?
g. There isn't one ounce of truth in his testimony.
h. What a monstrous spectacle she made of herself!
i. Don't ask questions; just do what you're told.
j. The wave curled, then crashed with a thundering roar.

Phrase and Sentence Force

The force of phrases within sentences varies considerably with regard to overall meaning. Skillful speakers use more force on important words and phrases and less force on unimportant material. The decrease in force of overall vocal output through selective emphasis can do much to relieve vocal abuse for the person with a voice problem.

---

[7] Nouns receive more emphasis than do pronouns. Adjectives generally receive more stress than do nouns when coupled. Adverbs generally receive more stress than verbs when coupled. Verbs generally receive more stress than auxiliary verbs. Prepositions, conjunctions, and articles are generally not stressed.

EXERCISE

Analyze the following sentences, underlining important words and phrases, before reading them aloud. Decrease force on the unmarked portions and increase force on the underlined material.

a. As I was saying before being interrupted, she envisions herself as the perennial ingenue.
b. After having seen all of the evidence, I'm really not too sure.
c. Without any more delays, let us get on with rehearsal.
d. It may be my imagination, but I thought I heard the door open.
e. By the way, if you plan to come out again in the spring, do let us know.
f. I would like to say, moreover, that the Greek playwrights were more imaginative, on the whole, than were the Roman dramatists.
g. Whether you agree with me or not is unimportant; I know the information is correct.
h. Just in case you miss the first signal, be sure you turn right at the second.
i. While Nero fiddled, Rome burned.
j. We live in deeds, not years; in thoughts, not breaths; in feelings, not in figures on a dial.

Sustained Force

Sustained force can be used to achieve emotional impact or speech climax. Because of the dramatic nature of this kind of emphasis, it must be used both sparingly and judiciously. Sustained force can be used to intensify the emotional impact of dramatic passages of prose or poetry. It is also very useful in achieving a powerful climax to a series of ideas or a theme. One must be aware that the demands on the laryngeal structures are at a maximum during this type of vocal delivery, and vocal strain is likely to occur. Unless the client has achieved a high level of vocal rehabilitation and has developed a strong voice, his use of sustained force should not be encouraged. There are times when a speaker may use sustained force on shorter segments of speech for additional emphasis, for example, "I don't know whose gloves you're talking about, but THESE ARE MINE."

EXERCISES

1. Use sustained force in performing the following sentences. Decide whether the entire sentence or only a portion should receive sustained force.
    a. Don't you dare come one step closer!
    b. How in heaven's name is it possible for you to forsake all your former beliefs?
    c. I cannot possibly accept your hedonistic philosophy.
    d. Don't tell me that you have forgotten again.
    e. O generation of vipers, how can you, being evil, speak good things?

2. The following sentences were used by speakers to achieve a high degree of climax through the use of sustained force.

   a. We have nothing to fear but fear itself!

—Franklin Delano Roosevelt

   b. Give me liberty, or give me death!   —Patrick Henry

   c. Ask not what your country can do for you—ask what you can do for your country.   —John F. Kennedy

   d. Friends! Romans! and Countrymen! Lend me your ears!

—Anthony, in William Shakespeare

   e. I have nothing to offer but blood, toil, tears, and sweat.

—Winston Churchill

3. Many speakers rely upon sustained force to achieve a high level of impact on longer segments of speech. Use sustained force judiciously on the two selections that follow.

   a. Brutus: Be patient till the last. Romans, countrymen, and lovers! hear me for my cause; and be silent, that you may hear: believe me for mine honor, and have respect to mine honor, that you may believe: censure me in your wisdom, and awake your senses, that you may the better judge. If there be any in this assembly, any dear friend of Caesar's, to him I say that Brutus' love to Caesar was no less than his. If then that friend demand why Brutus rose against Caesar, this is my answer: Not that I loved Caesar less, but that I loved Rome more. . . .

     —William Shakespeare, *The Tragedy of Julius Caesar*

   b. I have nothing to offer but blood, toil, tears, and sweat. . . . You ask, what is our policy? I will say, it is to wage war, by sea, land, and air, with all our might and with all the strength that God can give us; to wage war against a monstrous tyranny, never surpassed in the dark, lamentable catalogue of human crime. That is our policy. You ask, what is our aim? I can answer in one word: it is victory, victory at all costs, victory in spite of terror, victory, however long and hard the road may be; for without victory there is no survival.

     —Winston Churchill, Speech, May 13, 1940

Levels of Force

Many persons have to be taught how to adjust voice level to suit the occasion. At least five basic levels of force can be defined for typical speaking situations. It is possible to monitor one's loudness level through the sensory systems, namely, through auditory and PTK (proprioceptive-tactile-kinesthetic) feedback. Descriptions of the situations in which the basic levels would be used follow.

Level I:	Speaking easily to one or two people in quiet surroundings
Level II:	Speaking to a small group in a quiet living room
Level III:	Speaking to a group of 20 to 25 people in a typical class-room situation
Level IV:	Speaking to a group of 100 people in a large room or a small auditorium
Level V:	Speaking to a group in a medium to large auditorium

Factors that Influence Choice of Force Level

The *number of persons or size of audience* to whom you are speaking is one of the most important factors governing how much voice to use. Many speakers fail to recognize that listening can be fatiguing when the speaker's force level is low. The person with a voice problem should capitalize on a situation by reducing his force level when a higher level of force is not needed.

The *size of the room and space arrangement* require special considera-tion. If a conference room is long and narrow, a little more force is needed to project to the end of the table. Generally, the larger the room, the less help one will get from amplification through reverberation, as is true, for example, in the case of the shower room versus the classroom.

The *acoustical characteristics of the room or auditorium* have much to do with hearing. The dead room lacks reinforcement of sound energy, but the highly reverberant or noisy room can destroy much of the intelligibility of the speaker. A well-planned, acoustically treated room can do much to enhance speaker intelligibility.

The *availability of amplification* is of great importance in talking to large groups, particularly at Levels IV and V. Many speakers simply do not have enough force to talk to audiences at these levels, and amplification is therefore a prime requirement. The client should plan in advance to have amplification on hand if he is called upon frequently to talk to large audiences.

The *level of ambient noise present* is also an important factor to consider when adjusting voice level to a given speaking situation. For example, the level needed to talk to one person in quiet surroundings is markedly dif-ferent than that required for the same type of conversation at a noisy cock-tail party or on a busy street corner. Usually, the larger the audience and more reverberant the room, the greater the amount of force that is required to meet the demands of the situation.

Projection[8]

Very few people know how to project their voices properly, yet all of us are thrust into situations that demand the ultimate in terms of vocal output. To project one's voice improperly over a prolonged period of time can easily result in vocal fatigue and hoarseness. The breakdown of speakers' voices at political conventions is a good case in point. While projection requires increased breath control and relaxation, there are several other factors of vocal output that can be used to good effect. The following guidelines cover most of the main points to consider in projecting one's voice.

GUIDELINES

1. *Do not raise modal pitch level more than one or two half notes.* Speakers who raise their base pitch level more than one or two half notes in order to project their voices must increase tension to do so. Prolonged projection of one's voice at a higher-than-normal pitch level can easily result in fatigue and hoarseness. Remember, one's voice is fuller and more resonant at the optimum level, and to raise the base level unduly can easily reduce resonance, resulting in a loss of power.

2. *Concentrate upon relaxation of the mouth, throat, and larynx,* even though greater physical effort is exerted in projection. The average person tends to rely upon greater tension throughout the speech musculature to project his voice. A harsh or strident voice quality is a telltale sign that too much tension is present. Speakers who are successful in projecting their voices easily while using greater force are generally free from excessive tension throughout the speech musculature.

3. *Use shorter phrasing.* Projection requires shorter phrasing than does speech at lower levels of intensity. The shorter, more precise phrasing characteristic of successful projection makes a speaker easier to understand at a distance.

4. *Place stress upon the appropriate syllables and weaken the unstressed syllables by contrast.* The difference between stressed and unstressed syllables should increase as greater projection is required.

5. *Use more precise articulation.* Greater force demands precise articulation, particularly since supraglottic pressures increase during projection. A speaker is much easier to understand at a distance if he has appropriately precise articulation. Indistinct or inadequate articulation is greatly emphasized in projection and is to be avoided.

6. *Use greater force.* In order to be heard at a distance, greater force is usually necessary. Greater force should be based upon maximum use of resonance, including greater duration of vowels, diphthongs, glides, and

---

[8] Projection is a broad term referring to the utilization of a number of factors of speech in order to be heard better at a distance.

continuants. Higher levels of vocal output place greater demand upon laryngeal structures and functions than do lower levels of intensity.

7. *Use a slower rate of speaking and be sure to utilize pauses to maximum effect.* If all other factors of projection are observed, that is, greater duration, shorter phrasing, more precise articulation, and so on, speaking rate will inevitably be slower. Because projection involves more emphasis, pauses may be longer in duration and may occur more often. It is difficult to follow rapid speech at a distance.

EXERCISES

1. Perform the words that follow at five levels of loudness. Use good breath support, greater duration of sonorous speech sounds, good relaxation throughout the speech musculature, and do not raise your basic pitch level more than a note or two.

a. hi	f. fire	k. ball	p. no
b. halt	g. out	l. wait	q. shout
c. whoa	h. wow	m. boom	r. fine
d. well	i. zoom	n. go	s. done
e. how	j. ready	o. yes	t. rain

2. Using the instructions for Exercise 1, perform the following short sentences.

a. Where are you?	f. Ring the fire alarm!
b. Come over here!	g. I'm not going!
c. Who goes there?	h. Who said so?
d. Ball one!	i. No, no, I'll never go!
e. You're out!	j. It's high in the sky!

3. Theatre has long made use of the stage whisper—often occurring as "asides." In order to employ this technique successfully, one must have good breath supply, precise articulation, and ample projection. Now with these factors in mind, pretend you are projecting your voice to the back of a medium-sized auditorium—whisper.
   a. Hush! Here he comes!
   b. Should I tell him now; or should I wait?
   c. Sh-sh-sh! You mustn't talk out loud in church; the minister doesn't like it.
   d. Be real quiet; the fish won't bite when there is talking.
   e. Pst. Over here! Don't let them see you.

4. Read the following lines, using the five levels of projection for each. Follow the guidelines for projection carefully.
   a. O Captain! My Captain! Our fearful trip is done.
   b. Break, break, break, on thy cold gray stones, O sea.
   c. Awake! Awake! Ring the alarum bell!
   d. Gold! Gold! Gold! Gold! Bright and yellow, hard and cold. . . .
   e. Roll on, thou deep and dark blue Ocean, roll!

    f. This is no time for debate—this is the time for action!

    g. Free at last! free at last! thank God Almighty, we are free at last!

5. Often an entire portion of a speech or a selection will call for maximum projection. Practice the selections below, working for good projection and freedom from strain.

    a. Out of the night that covers me,
        Black as the Pit from pole to pole,
      I thank whatever gods may be
        For my unconquerable soul.

      In the fell clutch of circumstance
        I have not winced nor cried aloud.
      Under the bludgeonings of chance
        My head is bloody, but unbowed.

      Beyond this place of wrath and tears
        Looms but the Horror of the shade,
      And yet the menace of the years
        Finds, and shall find, me unafraid.

      It matters not how strait the gate,
        How charged with punishments the scroll,
      I am the master of my fate;
        I am the captain of my soul.
          —William Ernest Henley, "Invictus"

    b. Gold! Gold! Gold! Gold!
      Bright and yellow, hard and cold,
      Molten, graven, hammered, and rolled;
      Hard to get and heavy to hold;
      Hoarded, bartered, bought and sold,
      Stolen, borrowed, squandered, doled:
      Spurned by the young, but hugged by the old
      To the very verge of the church-yard mould;
      Gold! Gold! Gold! Gold!
      Good or bad a thousand-fold!
        How widely its agencies vary—
      To save—to ruin—to curse—to bless—
      As even its minted coins express,
      Now stamped with the image of good Queen Bess,
        And now of a Bloody Mary.
          —Thomas Hood, "Miss Kilmauseg and her Precious
            Leg: Her Misery"

    c. I met a traveller from an antique land
      Who said: "Two vast and trunkless legs of stone

Stand in the desert. Near them, on the sand,
Half sunk, a shattered visage lies, whose frown,
And wrinkled lip, and sneer of cold command,
Tell that its sculptor well those passions read
Which yet survive, stamped on these lifeless things,
The hand that mocked them, and the heart that fed;
And on the pedestal these words appear;
'My name is Ozymandias, king of kings;
Look on my works, ye Mighty, and despair!'
Nothing beside remains. Round the decay
Of that colossal wreck, boundless and bare,
The lone and level sands stretch far away."
    —Percy Bysshe Shelley, "Ozymandias"

d. Blow, winds, and crack your cheeks! rage! blow!
You cataracts and hurricanoes, spout
Till you have drench'd our steeples, drown'd the cocks!
You sulphurous and thought-executing fires,
Vaunt-couriers of oak-cleaving thunderbolts,
Singe my white head! And thou, all-shaking thunder,
Strike flat the thick rotundity o' the world!
Crack nature's moulds, all germens spill at once,
That make ingrateful man! . . .
Rumble thy bellyful! Spit, fire! spout, rain!
Nor rain, wind, thunder, fire, are my daughters:
I tax not you, you elements, with unkindness;
I never gave you kingdom, call'd you children,
You owe me no subscription: then let fall
Your horrible pleasure; here I stand, your slave,
A poor, infirm, weak, and despis'd old man;
But yet I call you servile ministers,
That will with two pernicious daughters join
Your high engender'd battles 'gainst a head
So old and white as this. O! O! 'tis foul!
    —from William Shakespeare, *The Tragedy of King Lear*

e. We shall not flag or fail. We shall go on to the end. We shall fight in France, we shall fight on the seas and oceans, we shall fight with growing strength in the air, we shall defend our Island, whatever the cost may be. We shall fight on the beaches, we shall fight on the landing grounds, we shall fight in the fields and in the streets, we shall fight in the hills; we shall never surrender, and even if, which I do not for a moment believe, this Island or a large part of it were subjugated and starving, then our empire beyond the seas, armed and guarded by the British Fleet, would carry on the struggle,

until, in God's good time, the New World, with all its power and
might, steps forth to the rescue and the liberation of the old.
—from Winston Churchill, Speech,
House of Commons, June 4, 1940

SELECTIONS FOR PRACTICE

1. The curfew tolls the knell of parting day,
   The lowing herd winds slowly o'er the lea,
The plowman homeward plods his weary way
   And leaves the world to darkness and to me.

Now fades the glimmering landscape on the sight,
   And all the air a solemn stillness holds,
Save where the beetle wheels his droning flight,
   And drowsy tinklings lull the distant folds;

Save that from yonder ivy-mantled tower
   The moping owl does to the moon complain
Of such as, wandering near her secret bower,
   Molest her ancient solitary reign.
         —from Thomas Gray, "Elegy Written in a
         Country Churchyard"

2. Here, where the world is quiet;
      Here, where all trouble seems
   Dead winds' and spent waves' riot
      In doubtful dreams of dreams;
   I watch the green field growing
   For reaping folk and sowing,
   For harvest-time and mowing,
      A sleepy world of streams.

   I am tired of tears and laughter,
      And men that laugh and weep,
   Of what may come hereafter
      For men that sow to reap;
   I am weary of days and hours,
   Blown buds of barren flowers,
   Desires and dreams and powers,
      And everything but sleep.
         —from Algernon Charles Swinburne,
         "The Garden of Proserpine"

3. Of all notable things on earth
   The queerest one is pride of birth,
      Among our "fierce Democracie"!

A bridge across a hundred years,
Without a prop to save it from sneers,—
Not even a couple of rotten Peers,—
A thing for laughter, fleers, and jeers,
   Is American aristocracy.

.   .   .

Depend upon it, my snobbish friend,
Your family thread you can't ascend,
Without good reason to apprehend
You may find it waxed at the farther end
   By some plebian vocation;
Or, worse than that, your boasted Line
May end in a loop of stronger twine,
   That plagued some worthy relation!
      —from John Godfrey Saxe,
        "The Proud Miss MacBride"

4. In May, when sea-winds pierced our soli-
       tudes,
  I found the fresh Rhodora in the woods,
  Spreading its leafless blooms in a damp
       nook,
  To please the desert and the sluggish brook.
  The purple petals, fallen in the pool,
  Made the black water with their beauty
       gay;
  Here might the red-bird come his plumes
       to cool,
  And court the flower that cheapens his
       array.
  Rhodora! if the sages ask thee why
  This charm is wasted on the earth and sky,
  Tell them, dear, that if eyes were made
       for seeing,
  Then Beauty is its own excuse for being:
  Why thou wert there, O rival of the rose!
  I never thought to ask, I never knew:
  But, in my simple ignorance, suppose
  The self-same Power that brought me
       there brought you.
        —from Ralph Waldo Emerson, "The Rhodora;
        On Being Asked Whence Is the Flower"

5. It was many and many a year ago,
    In a kingdom by the sea,
That a maiden there lived whom you may know
    By the name of Annabel Lee;
And this maiden she lived with no other thought
    Than to love and be loved by me.

I was a child and she was a child,
    In this kingdom by the sea,
But we loved with a love that was more than love—
    I and my Annabel Lee;
With a love that the wingèd seraphs of heaven
    Coveted her and me.

And this is the reason that, long ago,
    In this kingdom by the sea,
A wind blew out of a cloud, chilling
    My beautiful Annabel Lee;
So that her highborn kinsmen came
    And bore her away from me,
To shut her up in a sepulchre
    In this kingdom by the sea.
            —from Edgar Allan Poe, "Annabel Lee"

6. Build thee more stately mansions, O my
            soul,
            As the swift seasons roll!
            Leave thy low-vaulted past!
Let each new temple, nobler than the last,
Shut thee from heaven with a dome more
            vast,
            Till thou at length art free,
Leaving thine outgrown shell by life's un-
            resting sea.
            —from Oliver Wendell Holmes,
               "The Chambered Nautilus"

7. Three fishers went sailing out into the West,
    Out into the West as the sun went down;
Each thought on the woman who loved him the best;
    And the children stood watching them out of the town;
For men must work, and women must weep,
And there's little to earn, and many to keep,
    Though the harbour bar be moaning.

Three wives sat up in the light-house tower,
    And they trimm'd the lamps as the sun went down;

They look'd at the squall, and they look'd at the shower,
    And the night rack came rolling up ragged and brown!
But men must work, and women must weep,
Though storms be sudden, and waters deep,
    And the harbour bar be moaning.

Three corpses lay out on the shining sands
    In the morning gleam as the tide went down,
And the women are weeping and wringing their hands
    For those who will never come back to the town;
For men must work, and women must weep,
And the sooner it's over, the sooner to sleep—
    And good-bye to the bar and its moaning.
        —Charles Kingsley, "The Three Fishers"

8. Under the wide and starry sky,
Dig the grave and let me lie.
Glad did I live and gladly die,
And I laid me down with a will.

This be the verse you grave for me:
Here he lies where he longed to be;
Home is the sailor, home from sea,
    And the hunter home from the hill.
        —from Robert Louis Stevenson, "Requiem"

9. How do I love thee? Let me count the ways.
I love thee to the depth and breadth and height
My soul can reach, when feeling out of sight
For the ends of Being and ideal Grace.
I love thee to the level of everyday's
Most quiet need, by sun and candle-light.
I love thee freely, as men strive for Right;
I love thee purely, as they turn from Praise.
I love thee with the passion put to use
In my old griefs, and with my childhood's faith.
I love thee with a love I seemed to lose
With my lost saints,—I love with the breath,
Smiles, tears, of all my life!—and, if God choose,
I shall but love thee better after death.
        —from Elizabeth Barrett Browning,
          "Sonnets from the Portuguese, XLIII"

10. Swiftly walk o'er the western wave,
        Spirit of Night!
Out of the misty eastern cave,
Where, all the long and lone daylight,

Thou wovest dreams of joy and fear,
Which make thee terrible and dear—
      Swift be thy flight!

Wrap thy form in a mantle gray,
      Star-inwrought!
Blind with thine hair the eyes of Day;
Kiss her until she be wearied out,
Then wander o'er city, and sea, and land,
Touching all with thine opiate wand—
      Come, long-sought!

When I arose and saw the dawn,
      I sighed for thee;
When light rode high, and the dew was gone,
And noon lay heavy on flower and tree,
And the weary Day turned to his rest,
Lingering like an unloved guest,
      I sighed for thee.

Thy brother Death came, and cried,
      "Wouldst thou me?"
Thy sweet child Sleep, the filmy-eyed,
Murmured like a noontide bee,
"Shall I nestle near thy side?
Wouldst thou me?"—And I replied,
      "No, not thee!"
        —from Percy Bysshe Shelley, "To Night"

11. To myself, mountains are the beginning and the end of all natural scenery; in them, and in the forms of inferior landscape that lead to them, my affections are wholly bound up; and though I can look with happy admiration at the lowland flowers, and woods, and open skies, the happiness is tranquil and cold, like that of examining detached flowers in a conservatory, or reading a pleasant book; and if the scenery be resolutely level, insisting upon the declaration of its own flatness in all the detail of it . . . it appears to me like a prison, and I cannot long endure it. But the slightest rise and fall in the road—a mossy bank at the side of a crag of chalk, with brambles at its brow, overhanging it, a ripple over three or four stones in the stream by the bridge, above all, a wild bit of ferny ground under a fir or two, looking as if, possibly, one might see a hill if one got to the other side of the trees—will instantly give me intense delight, because the shadow, or the hope, of the hills is in them.
      —from John Ruskin, "Essays"

12. Vanity of vanities, saith the Preacher, vanity of vanities, all is vanity. What profit hath man of all his labour wherein he laboureth under the sun?

One generation goeth, and another generation cometh: and the earth abideth for ever. The sun also ariseth, and the sun goeth down, and hasteth to his place where he ariseth. The wind goeth toward the south, and turneth about unto the north; it turneth about continually in its course, and the wind returneth again to its circuits. All the rivers run into the sea, yet the sea is not full: unto the place whither the rivers go, thither they go again.

All things are full of weariness, man cannot utter it: the eye is not satisfied with seeing, nor the ear filled with hearing.

That which hath been is that which shall be; and that which hath been done is that which shall be done: and there is no new thing under the sun. Is there a thing whereof men say, See, this is new? It hath been already, in the ages which were before us.

There is no remembrance of the former generations; neither shall there be any remembrance of the later generations that are to come after.

  —from Ecclesiastes, the Bible

Relaxation

The pressures and tensions of our world have created a demanding environment in which we all must live. Inevitably, the economic, social and political demands upon the individual require constant adjustments, which all too often take the form of increased physical tension. The human voice characteristically reflects the varying degrees of tension we experience. Many clients seeking help for voice problems exhibit excessive tension throughout the speech mechanism. Today, most authorities agree that relaxation training should be included in voice rehabilitative programs for those who need it.

Rationale for Relaxation Instruction

1. *Certain types of clients need to free themselves from unwanted tension.* The person with a voice problem may have more tension throughout the vocal tract than does the person with a normal voice. This is generally true in passive postures as well as in active states.
2. *Good voice production requires the unhampered coordination of the muscles of phonation.* Excessive muscular tension is often present in both the intrinsic and extrinsic muscles of the larynx. Unwanted tension can interfere with the fine adjustments and coordination needed for producing a satisfactory laryngeal tone.
3. *Voice quality can be improved through relaxation.* Tension in the human resonating system, particularly in the texture of the walls of the pharyngeal and oral cavities, can contribute to inappropriate voice quality. This is especially true in the cases of harsh and strident voices.
4. *Relaxation prepares the individual for voice training.* Relaxation exer-

cises are often needed to reduce residual tension in the muscles used in voice in order to insure maximum efficiency in production.

5. *Relaxation must be taught.* A tense person generally does not respond readily when he is told simply to relax. He has to be taught to do it.

6. *Relaxation helps to break up old detrimental habits of tension during phonation.* Many voice cases need to acquire new habits of relaxation in order to break up old patterns of tension. It is generally true that if a client continues to meet life situations with his old habits of excessive tension, he will decrease the likelihood that he will be able to use the new behaviors he has acquired in the clinic.

7. *Relaxation is a powerful inhibitor of negative emotion.* Relaxation achieved through specific relaxation procedures can be used reciprocally to inhibit negative emotion. The treatment of voice disorders through systematic desensitization in stimulus situations has been used effectively by voice clinicians. Relaxation is typically used as the reciprocal inhibitor of negative emotion.

GUIDELINES

1. If required, relaxation procedures should be scheduled early in the training program.

2. Activities should be limited to a specific approach with a stated goal in training.

3. More time should be spent in relaxation procedures in the first few sessions, then decreased as the client gains control of the process.

4. In all approaches, make a definite assignment to practice procedures daily.

5. The client should rehearse all procedures in the clinic until he can do them by himself without prompting.

APPROACHES TO RELAXATION

Several different approaches to relaxation have been used by clinicians. Choice of approach often depends upon the goal of the training program. The wide range of procedures contained in this chapter far exceed the requirements for any one voice case; therefore, it is important that the clinician be thoroughly familiar with all approaches to relaxation in order to make a judicious choice for his client.

If relaxation is to be used as an inhibitor of negative emotion, the procedures for progressive relaxation, scene presentation, or hypnosis are typically used. If the client has difficulty in achieving relaxation by these approaches or does not want to participate in this type of procedure, the general and specific exercises may prove useful. The remainder of the relaxation procedures presented in this chapter are concerned with maintaining relaxation while engaged in activities.

PROGRESSIVE RELAXATION

Relaxation of a muscle has been defined by Jacobson as "the complete absence of all contractions."[1] His term, progressive relaxation, embraces a three-fold concept: (a) as a client works on a given muscle group, relaxation becomes deeper and deeper as the minutes go by; (b) for each new group of muscles relaxed, the groups previously worked on also relax; and (c) as the client practices daily, he progresses in relaxation, and the state is maintained automatically.

Jacobson stresses that it is important for the client to develop *muscle sense* as he is learning to relax. The term muscle sense is used to indicate the development of an inner awareness (kinesthetic and proprioceptive) of the state of tension remaining in the muscle group. The process of relaxing is mainly an attempt to rid oneself of *residual tension*, for in obtaining deeper and deeper states of relaxation, the tension in the muscle group abates. Frequently, a client will not be aware of the sites of tension and, with the aid of a clinician, must locate areas of unwanted residual tension. These areas are then scheduled for concentrated work, and the client practices deep relaxation until it has been established. Jacobson has found that the involuntary muscles of the body become relaxed as the voluntary muscle groups are freed from residual tension.

The principles of Jacobson's method of progressive relaxation have been used in speech and voice training since the 1930s. The procedures have been modified considerably to suit the needs of the client and the time factor of the clinical situation. The areas of concentration have been confined chiefly to the speech musculature. Instead of working for prolonged sessions to obtain deep relaxation in a given muscle group, short sessions stressing contrasts between tension and relaxation have been in common use by speech clinicians.

The use of progressive relaxation by Wolpe and others as a reciprocal inhibitor of negative emotion did much to restore the purpose of the Jacobson method, namely, achieving deep relaxation.[2] In order to serve as a reciprocal inhibitor, a general relaxation state must be achieved by the client of less than 15 sensation units of detection (suds) on a scale where 100 suds indicate the extreme of residual tension. This is a subjective scale based on 0 indicating no residual tension; 25 suds, quarter residual tension; 50 suds, half tension; and so forth. The degree of residual tension can be recorded by sensitive electronic equipment (i.e., electromyographic equipment). A base line of deep relaxation (less than 15 suds) can be established by the Jacobson method of progressive relaxation, by scene presentation, and by hypnosis.

---

[1] E. Jacobson, *You Must Relax* (New York: McGraw-Hill, 1962).
[2] J. Wolpe, A. Salter, and L. J. Reyna, *The Conditioning Therapies* (New York: Holt, Rinehart and Winston, 1964).

In voice training, progressive relaxation can be used in one of two ways: (a) to obtain relaxation deep enough to serve as an inhibitor to negative emotion, and (2) to obtain sufficient relaxation to free the speech musculature of enough tension in the regions of the larynx and pharynx for normal voice production.

PROCEDURES

After explaining the principles of progressive relaxation to the client, demonstrate the difference between muscle tension and relaxation. Use electronic equipment if available to monitor tension. About twenty minutes or more is needed to complete a full program. The client should spend thirty minutes to one hour every day practicing outside the clinic, which should speed up the acquisition of deep relaxation. Some clinicians prefer the client to work on deep relaxation of various muscle groups away from the clinic. The number of muscle groups can be reduced as skill in relaxation is acquired. Usually about six sessions are needed for clients to gain control of deep relaxation. The amount of time can be decreased to five minutes after the initial period of training. Be sure to include deep relaxation of the head and neck regions in all sessions. If it is possible for the client to practice relaxation procedures on his own ten minutes before the clinician commences working with him, valuable time can be devoted to other voice matters.

Progressive relaxation requires the client to become highly aware of the states of tension and relaxation in muscle groups. The following exercises are adapted from techniques commonly used in behavior therapy.

EXERCISES

1. Relaxation of the hands. Begin with the hands as follows:
   a. Settle comfortably in your chair.
   b. Clench your right fist, tighter, tighter.
   c. Now relax, allowing the fingers of your right hand to become more loose. Concentrate on relaxation for ten seconds.
   d. Repeat Steps b and c of tension and relaxation, attempting to increase the feeling of relaxation in your hand and fingers.
   e. Now clench both of your fists, tighter, tighter. Hold for more than five seconds.
   f. Now relax, deeper, deeper. Notice how the relaxation seems to extend to the rest of your body.

Exercise 1 can be done on any set of antagonistic muscles (i.e., those that work in opposition to each other), such as the extensor and flexor muscles of the arm. Usually, a program of relaxation for the entire body is given. The following areas are commonly explored. It is probably easiest to start with the hands or arms.

2. Relaxation of the arms
   a. Clench your fists, tighter, tighter; then relax.
   b. Tense the flexors and extensors of the arms. Relax; concentrate on the difference.

3. Relaxation of the head, neck, and shoulders
   a. Tense the muscles of your forehead and raise your eyebrows. Relax; feel the difference.
   b. Widen and tense the muscles of your eyes. Relax.
   c. Tense masseter muscles of your jaw (the chewing muscles). Relax.
   d. Tense tongue by pressing against the gum ridge of lower teeth. Relax.
   e. Tense the muscles involved in a pout, mouth closed. Relax.
   f. Tense the muscles of your neck by placing the palm of your hand against your forehead and pressing. Relax.
   g. Tense muscles of your neck by rolling your head straight back. Relax.
   h. Tense shoulders by an extreme shrug. Relax.
   i. Open your mouth and thrust your lower jaw forward under hard tension. Relax.
   j. Tense laryngeal muscles by impounding the airflow subglottally.

4. Relaxation of chest, stomach, and back
   a. Tense muscles of inhalation and exhalation. Relax.
   b. Tense muscles of upper rib cage. Relax.
   c. Tense lower abdominal muscles. Relax.
   d. Tense muscles of the upper legs and lower back. Relax.

5. Relaxation of legs and feet
   a. Tense muscles of the feet much the same way as clenching your fist. Relax.
   b. Flex and tense your toes and feet upward as far as you can go toward your shins. Relax.
   c. Tense all muscles above and below the knees. Relax.

6. A variation of these exercises, which the authors have used extensively, employs a more graded series of steps of tension and relaxation.
   a. Tense your fist, tighter, tighter. Hold clenched for ten seconds.
   b. Now relax. Feel the difference, which is extreme. Concentrate on the feeling of relaxation ten seconds.
   c. Tense your fist, but not as much. Hold the tension constant for ten seconds.
   d. Now relax. Feel the difference and try to obtain a greater feeling of relaxation—let the hand go limp, allowing the fingers to straighten. Concentrate on relaxation ten seconds.
   e. Close your fist lightly. Hold it for ten seconds. Concentrate on the feel in the muscles. Hold for ten seconds.
   f. Now relax your hand. More, more. Feel the difference in your hand.

Try to relax even further—let all the muscle fibres go. Hold for ten seconds.

g. Now close your eyes and pretend you are clenching your fist without actually doing so. Tighter, tighter. You should be able to feel some tension in the muscles. Hold for ten seconds.

h. Now relax. Deeper, deeper. Let it go, let it go.

The last step develops a "feel" for relaxation, and in a short time the client should be able to free specific muscle groups from tension as he gains complete control of his body.

SUGGESTION

There are several different ways of inducing relaxation by suggestion, namely, scene presentation, direct suggestion, and prehypnotic suggestion.

Presenting Scenes

The presentation of pleasurable scenes to a client is used extensively in behavior therapy to induce a sense of well-being and relaxation. The scene is often used as a means of reciprocally inhibiting negative emotion in the client. Two approaches to scene presentation are possible: (a) presentation of scenes for general relaxation, and (b) presentation of short scenes as the inhibitor of negative emotion in systematic desensitization in stimulus situation training.

Presentation of Scenes for General Relaxation

The clinician may elect to present a scene of his own choosing. The scenes should be tranquil rather than active. Use as many sensory details as possible in describing the scene (e.g., visual, auditory, kinesthetic, tactile, and olfactory), provided, of course, that they conjure up pleasant thoughts. Two scenes are presented in this section for your use. Make up others as suggested by the client.

In scene presentation for general relaxation, it is important to control external stimuli that may interfere with the client's thought processes, such as competing noises, visual distraction, or an unduly warm room. A comfortable chair, low-key lighting, and a quiet room are recommended. Many clinicians prefer to present the scenes from an adjacent room via a speaker system.

Relaxation is usually achieved in less time with scene presentation than with most other methods; therefore, scene presentation is used extensively in voice training programs. Approximately ten to twenty minutes are needed for the first session. The amount of time can be decreased as the client learns to "give himself over" to suggestion. A tape recording of the presentation can be used by the clinician to good effect; therefore, if the time and room are available, the client can listen to the tape and relax before the clinician arrives for the training session.

1. Have the client close his eyes and listen while you present the scene to him.

Close your eyes and rest. I want you to think about a little room, your own special room. You are sitting in a soft, comfortable chair. There is a large window looking out over a broad landscape. You are very happy in your room. Comfortable and relaxed. You can see a huge snow-capped peak in the distance. The snow sparkles in the sunshine. The slopes of the mountain are covered with a dense green forest. The tall pine trees on the ridges are silhouetted against the bright blue sky. Beautiful white clouds tower over the mountain, pushing up, up, up into the cobalt sky. It is beautiful and fresh. You can see a lake in front of the mountain. The lake is deep blue in the center but is jade green in the many bays and inlets. The sunlight glistens on the water. You can see a gull hovering over the lake, waiting, waiting, then he dives into the water. In front of the lake are flowers of all colors—red, cornflower blue, bright yellow. Now you can see a bed of roses, beautiful roses. You reach out and touch a deep, red rose that is perfect in form. You bend over and smell the aroma of the rose. You drink in the aroma. It is a lovely scent. You look upon the landscape, the mountain, the forest, the lake—it is a truly beautiful peaceful scene. You open your eyes. You are refreshed, relaxed, and happy.

2. Have the client close his eyes and listen while you present the following scene of "The Hill Country in Spring" to him.

Many artists have found that the hill country of south central Texas provides unusual scenes of great pastoral beauty in the Spring. The native bluebonnets blanket the gentle slopes of the hills. The oaks have just taken on their new leaves and stand resplendent in the bright sunshine. Their branches reach out in all directions and often run horizontally to the ground or bend down to the mulch of dead leaves lying beneath the tree. Here and there a thick clump of cactus commands a craggy prominence and the whole scene is alive with the sounds of nature—the cardinal as he calls to his mate, the bees as they hover over the spike-like clusters of the blue and white of the bluebonnets, and the myriad of tiny noises of insects. A soft blue and lavender haze seems to hover over the shallow valleys, bending away to the horizon. If you observe closely, you can see a trickle of fresh, clear water—one of 1100 springs that bubble forth from the rocks—as it spills over a sedge and wends its way through the glorious meadows to the Llano, the Medina, or the magnificent Guadalupe. As you contemplate the scene before you in all its tranquil beauty, the realization of something much greater than man, the meadows, the flowers, the insects and birds, the little rill, or even the stately oaks is there—serene, infinite, and eternal.

Presentation of Short Scenes

The presentation of short, pleasant scenes to inhibit negative emotion should be based upon information provided by the client. The clinician should ask the client, "What are some of the most pleasant scenes you can imagine?" Discuss the sensory details of these scenes sufficiently in order to present them to the client with accuracy. The clinician may only need to suggest some of the features of the scene, as the client's imagination should supply the rest. For example, if a child tells the clinician that getting an ice cream cone at the local ice cream parlor is his favorite memory, use it as the basis of a scene. Ask him to close his eyes and imagine the ice cream parlor, that he is walking up to the counter, making his choice, and so on. The scene need not last long, not more than twelve to fifteen seconds in systematic desensitization training. See Chapter 11 for a full discussion of the technique.

A second method of evoking pleasant memories for the client is to present slides of favorite places, people, or events by means of a slide projector and a screen. After presenting the picture, tell the client to close his eyes and imagine the scene as it was in real life.

Direct Suggestion

It is possible to make the client relax by direct suggestion. He is asked to sit in a comfortable chair (or lie in a supine position), close his eyes, and share in recreating the scenes that are presented to him. The client may also be told to relax various muscles by the clinician while in this position. The following dialogue is typical of this method of relaxation.

I want you to close your eyes and rest. You feel very comfortable now. I want you to think about the top of your head. It is warm—you can feel the blood flowing through the muscles. I want you to release all tension. It is warm and you are peaceful and happy. You feel the muscles of your forehead relax. Let them go, deeper, deeper. The blood flows through the muscles of your forehead, and you are comfortable and warm. Think about your eyes and relax. Let the tension go—more, more. You are very peaceful. The muscles of your cheeks and lips are relaxed. You can feel them getting heavier and heavier; let them go, deeper, deeper. You can feel the blood flow through your cheeks and lips and you are warm and comfortable. You are relaxing more deeply now. Now you can feel the muscles of your tongue and jaw relax. Let them go, more, more. You can feel the blood flowing through your tongue and jaw and you relax more deeply. Relax the muscles of your throat and larynx. You feel the flow of blood through the muscles of your neck and you are warm and comfortable. Let the muscles go, more, more. Relax the muscles of your shoulders and chest. Deeper, deeper. Let them go. You feel very relaxed now and peaceful.

Prehypnotic Suggestion

The following procedure may be used to induce a sense of deep, general relaxation in the client.

PROCEDURES

1. The client is seated in a comfortable chair. A reclining chair is our first preference. The clinician is seated nearby. The room may be darkened somewhat, although this is not entirely necessary. A large signet ring is suspended on a thread and is placed two to three feet from the client's eyes.
2. The ring is made to swing back and forth laterally.
3. The client is told to look at the ring as requested from time to time.
4. The clinician speaks to the client in a continuous monologue. His voice is reassuring, quiet, warm, soothing. The clinician begins his monologue.

I want you to look at the ring. (*Pause*) It is moving from side to side. Back and forth (*Ring moves in a lateral motion, voice synchronizes with ring*), back and forth. Your eyes feel a little tired as you watch the ring. Close your eyes. (*Pause*) When I say *one*, I want you to open your eyes and look at the ring again. Three, two, *one*. Back and forth, back and forth. Your eyelids feel a little heavy. You would like to close your eyes. Close your eyes. You feel very comfortable now. I want you to concentrate on the top of your head. It is warm—you are peaceful and happy. You can feel the muscles of your forehead relax. The blood flows through the muscles of your forehead, and you are comfortable and warm. Now I want you to think about your eyes and relax. Your eyes are at ease. You are very peaceful. When I say *one* I want you to look at the ring again. Three, two, *one*. Open your eyes. The ring is moving back and forth, back and forth. Your eyelids are very heavy and you want to close your eyes. (*Pause*) Close your eyes. (*Pause*) The muscles of your cheeks and lips are relaxed. You can feel the flow of blood through the muscles. They are heavy and relaxed. (*Pause*) You feel warm and comfortable. You are relaxing more deeply now. When I say *one*, I want you to open your eyes, but only for an instant, then close them. *One*. That's right—close your eyes. You are glad to close your eyes. You are getting sleepy, now. You can feel the muscles of your jaw and tongue relax. The warm blood flows through your muscles and you are comfortable. You are peaceful and happy. Relax the muscles of your neck and shoulders, deeper, deeper. You feel warm and peaceful. Content. You are very relaxed and sleepy now. I want you to open your eyes when I say *one*, but only for an instant, then close them immediately. Your eyelids are very heavy now and you don't want to open your eyes. *One*. Fine. Relax your shoulders and chest. Deeper, deeper. Let them go. You are very warm and comfortable.

I want you to think about a little room, deep down inside of you. It is a lovely room. You are sitting in a soft, comfortable chair. There is a large window that you can see out over a broad scene. You are very happy in your room. Comfortable and relaxed. You look out of the window and you see a snow-capped peak. It is beautiful. The slopes are covered with tall pine trees. Beautiful white clouds tower over the mountain. The sky is a cobalt blue. It is a lovely sight. In front of the mountain is a sparkling, clear lake. The sunlight glistens on the water. The water is a deep blue. There is a field of flowers just outside the window. Flowers of all colors, red, yellow, white—they are beautiful. You bend over and smell the aroma of a deep, red, rose. You drink in the aroma. (*Pause*) When I say *one* I want you to open your eyes, *refreshed*, relaxed, and happy. Three, two, *one*; open your eyes.

GENERAL-TO-SPECIFIC RELAXATION

If a general-to-specific approach to relaxation is used, the clinician is free to choose from a wide range of exercises. Naturally, he should be selective about those included in the program, since many of the exercises included in this section tend to duplicate each other in terms of the results achieved. Approximately ten minutes should be all that is required for this type of exercise. Start work on the larger, general exercises, such as the elephant walk, then proceed to the specific exercises involving both the head and neck muscles (nonphonatory). Finally, do those exercises that involve the use of voice. It is important to drill the client on all of these exercises until he can do them well on his own. Assignments should be made for practice away from the clinic. After several sessions (involving success, of course), the amount of time devoted to this type of relaxation can be reduced.

GENERAL RELAXATION EXERCISES

1. Elephant walk. Let your body flop over at the waist like a rag doll. Let your arms be the elephant's trunk. Now move forward head down and arms loose, swaying your torso from side to side. Attempt to loosen the muscles of your spine, rib cage, and shoulders. Walk at least ten feet.

2. Take a deep breath and yawn, stretching your arms and upper body like a giant cat. S-t-r-e-t-c-h.

3. Standing erect with your feet parted, drop your head on your chest. Now, slump your shoulders forward in an arch. Next, drop your head, shoulders, and body over at the waist. Gently shake your upper body loose from left to right and back again. Repeat.

SPECIFIC RELAXATION EXERCISES

These exercises, which loosen the muscles of the head and neck, may be done either sitting or standing.

1. Let your head drop forward of its own weight to your chest. Lift your head slowly back to its original position. Repeat two or three times.

2. Move your head backward (mouth closed) until your chin is as far back as you can go. Now stretch the muscles in the front of the neck—slowly. Repeat.

3. Turn your chin and head slowly to the right shoulder. When you have reached the limit of this extension, slowly stretch a bit farther, looking over your shoulder if you can. Do not turn your body. Repeat.

4. Repeat Exercise 3 to the left shoulder.

5. Drop your head forward on your chest, then slowly rotate it to the right in a complete circle. Attempt to relax all muscles in the head and shoulders that are not needed for this activity. Repeat. Reverse the direction of rotation by circling your head to the left. Go slowly. If you complete a full rotation in less than 12 seconds, you are going too fast. Note: Fast or jerky movements might easily lead to a pinched nerve and subsequent discomfort.

6. A second version of Exercise 5 is to move the shoulders in a circle that permits the head to follow loosely in the same orbit. Avoid speed and excess tension.

7. If you feel energetic and are limber enough, Exercise 5 can be extended to the entire body by rolling at the waist, letting the arms and upper torso follow loosely in a state of complete relaxation.

8. Drop your head to your chest. Let your jaw fall slack. Now gently shake your jaw loose, letting your lips and facial muscles go limp. Repeat, shaking gently until you achieve freedom from tension and rigidity.

9. Tense your jaw and neck muscles, tighter, tighter (for ten seconds). Now relax your neck and jaw as much as you can for ten seconds. Repeat, attempting with each effort to achieve a deeper feeling of relaxation.

10. Loosen and relax the jaw muscles by whispering (a whisper is preferable to normal speaking tones at this stage of training) the following syllable chains, involving the phonemes [ɑ] or [ʌ] in final position.

     a. wah-wah-wah-wah-wah-wah-wah-wah-wah-wah [ɑ]
     b. wuh-wuh-wuh-wuh-wuh-wuh-wuh-wuh-wuh-wuh [ʌ]
     c. yah-yah-yah-yah-yah-yah-yah-yah-yah-yah [ɑ]
     d. yuh-yuh-yuh-yuh-yuh-yuh-yuh-yuh-yuh-yuh [ʌ]
     e. shah-shah-shah-shah-shah-shah-shah-shah-shah [ɑ]
     f. shuh-shuh-shuh-shuh-shuh-shuh-shuh-shuh-shuh [ʌ]
     g. bah-bah-bah-bah-bah-bah-bah-bah-bah-bah [ɑ]
     h. buh-buh-buh-buh-buh-buh-buh-buh-buh-buh [ʌ]

11. Press the tip of the tongue against the roof of the mouth firmly for ten seconds. Release the pressure and relax the tongue ten seconds. Repeat, attempting to get greater relaxation with each successive trial.
12. A ballet dancer limbers up her hands by gently shaking them loose. With this concept in mind, bend over at the waist, letting your tongue and jaw hang loosely. Gently shake your head. Repeat.

THROAT RELAXATION EXERCISES

1. Attempt several stages of yawning.
   a. First, gently.
   b. More deeply.
   c. Yawn vigorously, closing your eyes and stretching the muscles of your mouth and throat.
2. Inhale, effecting a gentle yawn, then sigh *ah* in a prolonged, breathy downglide. Repeat.
3. Inhale deeply. Now sigh *ah* in a relaxed, breathy manner.
4. Attempt to develop an awareness of the *feel* of throat relaxation in the following sequence.
   a. Inhale slowly and deeply, then sigh *ah*. Concentrate upon the kinesthetic sensation of both inhalation and exhalation while you are performing.
   b. Close your eyes and attempt to recall the kinesthetic experience of this event.
   c. Repeat the exercise five times.

EXERCISE FOR RELAXATION WHILE LYING DOWN

1. Relaxation is often more readily achieved while lying in a supine position, particularly if the client is noticeably tense or inflexible. Ask him to lie down on his back with his arms folded comfortably on his chest. Most of the skeletal muscles should be inactive as they are not needed to support the body nor are they involved in physical activity. Ask the client to close his eyes.
2. Several variations of Exercise 1 are possible:
   a. Quietly describe a pastoral scene to the subject. Use the selection, "The Hill Country in Spring," p. 118.
   b. Play soothing music for the client and ask him to think pleasant

thoughts. Keep the volume level low. You may also darken the room somewhat to aid in reducing external visual stimuli.

c. Ask the client to think about pleasant experiences in his life. After he has been doing this for two or three minutes, observe his respiration; it should deepen considerably and cycle more slowly. Also, observe facial muscles, and other muscle groups for unwanted activity.

d. Use the progressive relaxation exercises found earlier in this chapter.

3. Engage the client in a quiet discussion to determine the state of relaxation of his muscles. Review the muscle groups systematically.

EXERCISES FOR RELAXATION WHILE ENGAGED IN ACTIVITIES

After relaxation has been achieved in the supine position, the client should be taught to relax in a variety of activities. These exercises should be included in *all* types of relaxation approaches.

1. Have the client maintain good posture and relaxation while reading a book in a comfortable chair. The spine should be straight and the book should be held directly in front of and below the eyes. Those muscles that are not involved in this posture should be normally relaxed.

2. Using the same chair, have the client maintain appropriate posture and good relaxation while engaging in a quiet conversation.

3. Have the client sit at a desk and write (a typical letter to a friend will do). Maintain good posture and relaxation.

4. In the same setting as in Exercise 3, have the client engage in a simulated telephone conversation. Check the degree of relaxation by observing various muscles and by inquiry.

5. Have the client stand and relax while listening to conversation.

6. Engage the client in conversation while he is under instructions to maintain good relaxation and posture.

7. Obtain information from the client with regard to typical speech situations that occur in his life regularly and are difficult for him to relax in. These situations may be recreated and rehearsed under conditions of control within the training situation.

EXERCISES FOR RELAXATION AND PHONATION

1. Combine relaxation and phonation in the following situations:
   a. Inhale and sigh, *ah*   [ɑ]
   b. Inhale and sigh, *aw*   [ɔ]
   c. Inhale and sigh, *oh*   [oʊ]
   d. Inhale and sigh, *I*   [aɪ]
   e. Inhale and sigh, *uh*   [ʌ]

2. Relax your mouth and throat muscles (think of a yawn), inhale, then say the following words one at a time:

a. father	f. straw	k. old	p. my	u. up
b. arbor	g. cause	l. road	q. sigh	v. usher
c. almond	h. autumn	m. grow	r. shy	w. supper
d. olive	i. awful	n. code	s. nigh	x. thunder
e. balm	j. law	o. open	t. bright	y. oven

3. Use the same procedure as in Exercise 2 with the following phrases, maintaining good relaxation throughout:
   a. our father's car
   b. the winding old road
   c. the blowing snow
   d. the code of the law
   e. the autumn leaves
   f. from the almond tree
   g. for many of them
   h. to his shy brother
   i. for the arbor over there
   j. eating his supper by the fire

4. Use the same procedure for the following sentences, maintaining good relaxation:
   a. The cold gray dawn ushered in a new day.
   b. "Bah," quote grandpa, as his car hit the boulder hidden in the snow on the road.
   c. The rainbow's end and its pot of gold have eluded fortune hunters for time untold.
   d. Jim Carson wondered how much damage the fire had done.
   e. Flaws in the law are sought by probing lawyers.
   f. Grandpa gave grandma a lot of flak when she burned their contribution to the potluck supper.
   g. Poetic psalms act as balm to calm our troubled hearts.
   h. The hawk caught a toad in his sharp claws.
   i. Much trouble was averted by withdrawing the army early the next morning.
   j. The artist's cartoon was auctioned for a fortune.

5. Try the following words, attempting to get more jaw movement on the vowel in each succeeding word: *see, sit, say, sat, saw, psalm.*

6. Maintain good relaxation of the mouth, throat, and larynx as you babble nonsense syllable chains softly. Strive for a slightly breathy quality to alleviate laryngeal tension. Repeat several times, varying the pitch and intensity, but avoid volume above low conversational level and high pitch levels above the midpoint in your range.

7. In attempting to relax the speech musculature, reduce normal tensions and pressures to a point where you are lazily drawling out your words. Use the following practice sentences:
   a. A fine spray remained after the wave had crashed on the reef.
   b. My father is the strongest man in town.
   c. The gull hovered over the surf for an instant, then plunged sharply into the water.
   d. The cable car climbed slowly up the hill.
   e. Can you tell me how to get to 444 Fourth street?

f. I tell you, Jellycoat, that's the funniest thing I've seen in years.
g. "Not through the Iron Duke," he cried, as he played his king of spades.
h. Autumn's haze hung over the sprawling valley.
i. The song of the open road always beckons to me when the wild geese fly.
j. The wave's spume caught me unawares.

8

Breath
Control for Voice

Whether or not breathing exercises should be included in the rehabilitation program is a matter of debate. As with training in relaxation, there are those who believe that since breathing is a "natural process," or biological function, it does not have to be taught. Furthermore, those who are reluctant to work on breathing for voice *per se* point out that very little more air is needed for speech than for life purposes and that, under normal circumstances, the organism will regulate airflow *naturally*. Adherents of the chewing method point out that as normal chewing functions are instituted and combined with speech, respiration returns to within normal limits for adequate voice.

There are many adjustments in breath control necessary for maintaining or changing subglottic air pressure in normal voice production, including those required for pitch and loudness shifts. To assume that the client has adequate control or had adequate control before developing a voice problem is an error. This does not imply that all clients require training in breathing, for such is not the case. It is entirely possible that some clients will demonstrate breathing habits for voice that are within normal limits; such clients do not require more than passing reminders to utilize this ability both in the clinic and throughout the day. The authors tend to embrace the point of view that breathing procedures should be considered when they are clearly indicated, but should not be undertaken when the client demonstrates adequate respiratory habits for voice and speech.

GUIDELINES FOR TEACHING BREATH CONTROL

1. Have the client inhale through the mouth instead of the nose. In almost all breathing for voice, inhalation is through the mouth, particularly since it is easier and faster.

2. Monitor airflow by listening to the air rushing through the partially closed lips. Have the client purse his lips in order to partially occlude the passageway. This will permit both the clinician and the client to monitor the speed, amount, and duration of inhalation and exhalation on nonvocal depth, center, and "control" exercises.

3. Do not place too much emphasis on depth of breathing. Breathing for voice should be natural and does not require an inordinate amount of air. The average inhalation for voice is only slightly deeper than for life purposes. Control is the important factor.

4. Work from a given base line of residual air. It is not necessary to use the exhalatory reserve in most exercises.

5. Work for central control of breathing; that is, using medial-dia-phragmatic abdominal breathing. Central control will tend to reduce the need for upper thoracic control (expansion of upper rib cage) and will do much toward eliminating unwanted tension in the neck. Eventually, control will be much more sensitive and effective.

6. Monitor breathing by observing the movements visually and feeling the movements through the PTK (proprioceptive-tactile-kinesthetic) senses. The client will eventually learn to associate the memory of correct movements through the sensory feedback loop.

7. Attempt to improve upon the client's best performance in order to increase his ability to control the respiratory processes.

8. Care should be observed when combining breathing exercises with voice. Since the client may not have worked on phonation, vocalization may prove difficult for him. Therefore, it is best to work with lower levels of intensity since they are less demanding on the structures involved. It may also be wise to instruct the client to use a slightly breathy voice to reduce vocal effort.

9. Breath control exercises for greater force should not be undertaken until the client has demonstrated good phonatory habits. Rehearsal under conditions of poor phonation could be harmful.

10. Have the client perform all assigned exercises without prompting from the clinician. This is especially important because of the need to practice away from the clinic.

CENTRAL CONTROL OF BREATHING

EXERCISES

Perform the following exercises without utilizing voice.

1. Sitting in a straight-backed chair, bend over and grasp the front legs of the chair near the top. Keep the soles of your feet on the floor. Inhale slowly as far as you can go. Observe the expansion in the lower rib cage and abdominal areas as you are inhaling. Repeat, attempting to

increase the amount of inhalation. Note: In this position it is almost impossible to expand your rib cage by lifting your shoulders.

2. While either sitting or standing, place one hand to one side slightly above the hip. Place the other hand on your abdominal wall just below the sternum; be sure that your thumb is over the lower margin of the rib cage while your fingers are extended forward and slightly downward over your abdomen. Spread your fingers slightly in order to feel any movement in the abdominal area. Inhale slowly through your mouth. Try to keep your upper rib cage from expanding or rising. Observe and feel the frontal expansion of the abdomen; note also the lateral movements of the ribs. If the rib action does not take place, attempt to introduce this movement on the next trial. Attempt to increase the depth of inhalation with each successive trial.

3. With your hands in the same position as in Exercise 2, inhale, then slowly exhale, noting the action of the abdominal wall and the lateral rib cage. Prolong the exhalatory part of the cycle by squeezing out the last bit of breath. Next, increase the depth of inhalation, which will permit a longer period of exhalation. Lastly, attempt to speed up the inhalatory part of the cycle but maintain the same depth, then try to increase the exhalatory part of the cycle in successive trials. Study the interaction between the diaphragm, the abdominals, and the intercostals as you are performing this exercise.

4. You may explore your breathing center and capacity by lying on your back. Breathe regularly, easily, deeply. Note that in this position it is difficult to move the shoulders and upper chest; thus, it is quite likely that abdominal (or central) breathing is taking place. Try to increase your capacity. Vary the cycle of inhalation and exhalation much the same as you did in Exercise 3.

5. Any device that can measure the amount of expansion laterally and frontally can be put to good use to demonstrate central control to the client. The following techniques are suggested.

   a. Use a tailor's soft tape measure to check expansion in terms of inches and fractions of inches. Place the tape over the areas of maximum expansion, that is, the lower margins of the rib cage and the upper abdominal wall. Overlap the tape in front and measure your body before inhalation. Inhale slowly and observe the expansion on the tape. When you have reached your limit, take a measurement. Subtract the first measurement from the second; the difference is the amount of expansion from a base line position. Repeat the exercise, attempting to better your record.

   b. A cord or belt may be used if you don't have a soft tape measure. Place the cord over the areas of maximum expansion and make a reference mark on the overlapped cord. Inhale and note how far the reference mark has moved from its original position. Measure the amount expanded on a straight ruler. Repeat, attempting to improve upon your best record.

c. Instruments such as a wet spirometer can be used to measure the amount of air inhaled in cubic centimeters. Note: If you are seeking *central* control, avoid upper chest and clavicular breathing in all of these exercises.

6. Stand in an erect position using good posture. Press a book against your abdominal wall. Inhale slowly without raising your shoulders or upper chest. Observe the forward movement of the book. Repeat, attempting to achieve greater forward movement of the book. Note: This exercise does not account for lateral movement.

7. A classic version of Exercise 6 is as follows: Lie in a supine position (on your back) on a rug or firm bed. Place several heavy books on your abdomen. Raise the books by slowly inhaling. Balance the books and do not let them fall. Attempt to increase the amount you can raise the books. Many professional performers—singers, actors, and the like—have used this exercise not only to locate the center of breathing but also to strengthen the abdominal muscles by adding more books to the pile.

8. Several forms of popular physical exercise will help to develop natural breathing habits and markedly increase capacity. Exercises such as walking, jogging, running in place, cycling, swimming, and rowing are among the best forms of this type of activity.

a. Kenneth Cooper, M.D., in his book, *The New Aerobics*, advocates use of all these exercises (except rowing) as a means of gaining 100 percent physical fitness. The purpose of walking, jogging, cycling, or swimming is to put pressure on the respiratory system to supply oxygen to the bloodstream to meet the demands of the muscles involved in the activity. The subject progresses through a carefully graded series of exercise schedules leading to 100 percent fitness, usually met after sixteen weeks of activity. A system of points is assigned to the number of minutes involved and the rate of the activity per minute. Read *New Aerobics* carefully before embarking on this type of respiratory exercise.

b. Using a rowing machine is perhaps one of the best methods of strengthening the abdominal muscles and increasing exhalatory power. A famous operatic baritone once remarked that he had "rowed across the United States" while preparing for a New York concert.

EXERCISES

Perform the following exercises to develop central breath control while vocalizing.

1. Place one hand to one side just above the hip and the other on your abdominal wall just below the sternum; be sure that your fingers are spread slightly to cover both the lower rib cage and the abdomen. Inhale deeply, but try to limit the expansion to the central area. Then count out loud slowly up to five. Keep the pitch and intensity levels constant. Avoid fading on the final numbers in the count.

2. Repeat, only this time increase the count to six. Continue in this manner until you reach the count of ten. Observe as well as feel the expansion and contraction of the respiratory system.

3. Repeat Exercise 1, using counts of 12, 15, 18, 21, 24, 27, and 30. Try to work within your capacity to count evenly and smoothly up to a given number without forcing. Avoid squeezing out your exhalatory reserve air. Go on to a higher level as you increase inhalation. Again, try to concentrate on expansion of the central area and attempt to minimize upper chest expansion.

4. Sustain various speech sounds over time. Use a watch with a second hand to time the performance. Keep pitch and intensity levels constant. Concentrate on central control and avoid squeezing out the air during the last few seconds.

    a. Inhale, then exhale, sustaining *ah* [ɑ] while monitoring central control and time.

    b. Sustain the following vowels in successive trials, monitoring both central control and time. Keep a record to refer back to on future trials. Try to better your best performance.

[i]	as in *see*	[u]	as in *who*
[ɛ]	as in *let*	[o]	as in *obey*
[æ]	as in *can*	[ɔ]	as in *law*
[ʌ]	as in *run*	[ɑ]	as in *father*

    c. Sustain the following consonants: [s, ʃ, f, m, l, z, h]. Monitor both time and central control.

5. Practice speaking materials of a serial nature, observing central control.

    a. a b c d e f g h i j k l m n o p q r s t u v w x y z (continue on to a, b, c, etc.).

    b. Monday, Tuesday, Wednesday, Thursday, Friday, Saturday, Sunday, Monday, etc.

    c. January, February, March, April, May, June, July, August, September, October, November, December, January, February, etc.

6. Read the following sentences, keeping pitch and intensity relatively uniform. How far were you able to read comfortably? Mark the last word you reached and repeat. Attempt to improve on your record.

    a. When the three boys reached the promontory, they were able to see the vast expanse of ocean, lying before them in all its great panorama of color, movement, and sea life, resembling, as Tim recalled later, a painting by the great American seascape artist, Winslow Homer, who would have enjoyed painting the very scene before the young adventurer.

b. The thick brown cloud began to settle over the city as evening drew on, with no promise of respite from the blast furnaces of the three big steel companies ringing the western edge of the metropolis, whose tall stacks continued to belch forth their yellow-brown columns of smoke curling up into the polluted air above, as if urging the clouds to move over to make room for more.

c. Early in the morning as the eastern sky was firing up and the clouds began to take on the myriad rosy hues of the slanting rays of the sun, we slowly wended our way through the heavy jungle-like growth of ferns, coconut palms, and banana trees so typical of the semi-tropical vegetation of the San Blas area en route to Mazatlan—our trailer heavily laden with enough supplies to last the three months of our vacation.

7. Lying on your back, place four or five heavy books on your abdomen. Repeat Exercises 1–6 in this series. You may increase the weight to add greater difficulty to the exercises. Concentrate on central breath control.

DEPTH OF BREATHING

EXERCISES FOR DEPTH OF BREATHING

1. This "cycle of breathing" exercise is valuable in developing greater sensitivity of control of breath as well as increasing capacity, or the amount of available air.

a. Inhale slowly (five seconds) over a silent count of six. Draw in the air evenly; purse your lips so that you can monitor airflow amount by listening to the rush of air.

b. Hold the air in your lungs *without closing your glottis* for a silent count of six.

c. Exhale slowly over a silent count of six. Keep the airflow even and be sure you have exhaled no more or less than the amount inhaled in Step a.

d. Hold in the exhaled position for a silent count of six. Be sure to keep your glottis open.

e. Repeat Steps a–d two more times in a continuous sequence. Note that the muscles of inhalation are used to maintain the respiratory system in the hold position in Step b, while the muscles of exhalation are held in contraction to maintain the hold position in Step d.

2. Exercise 1 may be extended in two ways to increase control and capacity.

a. Increase the count to seven, then to eight. Be sure that the speed of counting remains constant.

b. Synchronize the taking of steps with the count:

(1) Walk six steps while inhaling, then turn around. (The steps can be taken in one direction if there is enough room. Turning is suggested if the exercise must be performed in a confined space.)

(2) Walk back six steps while holding your breath with the glottis open, then turn around.

(3) Walk six steps while exhaling, then turn around.

(4) Walk six steps while holding the glottis open, but do not inhale. Repeat the cycle. Increase the count to seven, then eight. Walking during the silent count puts additional pressure and demand on the respiratory system and develops greater control. Step b is easily adapted to outside practice; the cycles can be done walking to a daily destination, such as school or work.

3. This exercise is good for developing depth of breathing.

a. Inhale to one-third of your total capacity. Release a small amount of air but not more than about one-fourth of what you just inhaled. Hold for three seconds but do not close your glottis—use your muscles of inhalation to hold it.

b. Inhale to two-thirds of your total capacity and release a small amount of air. Hold for three seconds. Again, do not close the glottis.

c. Now inhale to your total capacity, only this time do not release any air and hold your breath with the muscles of inhalation. Do not close your glottis. Hold for three seconds and release. On this step you will need to expand your upper chest for maximum capacity.

d. Repeat this exercise one more time. *Caution: do not do this exercise more than twice, as you can easily overoxygenate your blood stream and become dizzy.*

EXERCISES FOR COMBINING DEPTH AND CONTROL

1. Perform the following number chains, working for ease and comfort of breathing. Monitor the airflow both on inhalation and exhalation in terms of the PTK (proprioceptive-tactile-kinesthetic) feedback systems. You may use a slightly breathy quality, which will tend to demand greater supply and control. Perform odd- and random-numbered sequences as smoothly as the first sequence.

a. 1 - 2 - 3 - 4 - 5
b. 1 - 3 - 5 - 2 - 4
c. 1 - 3 - 5 - 7 - 2 - 4 - 6
d. 1 - 3 - 5 - 7 - 9 - 2 - 4 - 6 - 8
e. 1 - 4 - 7 - 6 - 3

    f.   3 - 8 - 9 - 5 - 6 - 4 - 2

    g.   7 - 4 - 8 - 9 - 6 - 1 - 3 - 2 - 5

2. Practice the following sentences, attempting to obtain adequate depth of breathing. Also, maintain good control over the outgoing airflow. Each of these sentences should be done on one continuous exhalation.

    a.   There is an inner world of beauty available to all.

    b.   Loud blasts of noise have been known to raise blood pressure.

    c.   Man's avarice and greed have resulted in pollution of the skies, the streams, the countryside, and seas.

    d.   The reading room of the main library, Ruth recalled later, was the most peaceful place on the campus.

    e.   The bulldozer was equipped with a steel probe that made it possible for Rex to unload the heavy sewer pipes from the truck.

BREATH CONTROL AND WASTAGE OF AIR

Many persons with a limited breath supply waste air needlessly during speech. This is particularly noticeable on one class of sounds, the voiceless fricatives—[f], [θ], [s], [ʃ], and [h]. If the quality of the voice remains the same while performing the exercises that follow, increasing intensity and duration of the sounds will require more breath supply. If intensity or duration of sounds is decreased while reading, less breath supply for given breath groups will be needed. Review the section on hypovalvular phonation in Chapter 4 before doing the following exercises.

EXERCISES

1. As a base line, prolong [f] holding the intensity constant and noting time in seconds to exhaust a normal inhalation. Do the same for [θ], [s], [ʃ], and [h]. Now repeat the series, first using low intensity and noting the time lapse per exhalation, and second using high intensity (more than on the first trial). Study the differences in time for each of the sounds at the three levels of intensity.

2. Vary the intensity and duration of [f], [θ], [s], [ʃ], and [h] in the following word chains.

    a.   fee - foe - fie - fey - fume - fan - fun - feign - fin - farm   [f]

    b.   thin - thick - thigh - thumb - think - thought - three - thank - thirty - thug   [θ]

    c.   see - sat - saw - sew - same - sue - sigh - save - sign - soil   [s]

    d.   she - shall - show - shake - sharp - shine - shoal - ship - shoe - shape [ʃ]

    e.   hoe - high - hey - how - home - hero - health - hat - ham - hail   [h]

3. Perform the following word pairs, allowing wastage on the first word but demonstrating conservation of air and normal production on the second word.

a. fun-fun fine-fine fat-fat fame-fame fin-fin   [f]
b. thick-thick thin-thin three-three through-through thatch-thatch   [θ[
c. soup-soup soap-soap sigh-sigh soar-soar sack-sack   [s]
d. shine-shine sure-sure shade-shade sheen-sheen shoal-shoal   [ʃ]
e. heart-heart heed-heed hence-hence hilt-hilt have-have   [h]

4. The following sentences contain many voiceless fricatives. Practice them in two ways, first demonstrating wastage, and second demonstrating good control of duration and intensity. Note the difference in air consumption.

a. Surely Sue should heed the heart's desire.
b. The ham was sliced both thick and thin.
c. The swallow soared through the starlit sky.
d. Sally's split pea soup was scalded.
e. The shore was slightly shaded by shiny, silvery sycamores.
f. Harold's shoeshine stand should net him a handsome profit.
g. The hydroplane cannot soar high in the sky, but it can skim over the sea.
h. She thought that it was fun to sail in the shipshape four-masted schooner.
i. Forty-four thousand three hundred and thirty-three sailors rise and shine to his bugle.
j. Fat Fanny ate soup until she shed forty-three pounds and thirteen ounces.

Lack of Breath Support on Phrases and Sentences

Three phenomena may be associated with lack of breath support at the ends of phrases or sentences: (a) the intensity diminishes noticeably toward the ends of the phrases or sentences, (b) tension develops in both the laryngeal and respiratory muscles in attempting to squeeze out more air to maintain voice, and (c) pitch breaks or glottal fry may occur as the airflow decreases below a level of tonal support.

EXERCISE

Read the following selections and analyze the results. A tape recorder should be used in studying the results of the reading. Mark the places where the voice fades or breaks. Repeat, attempting to eliminate faulty breath support.

a. Kaskaskia, once the commercial "queen of the West," the first capital city of Illinois, the seat of government during territorial days, and one of the principal settlements of the French, is gone now—long ago tumbled into the swirling flood-swollen waters of the Mississippi, and all that remains is an island and relics—a bell, a church, a cemetery. The prophecy and curse of an Algonquin Indian, angered by the French

settlement, was fulfilled. "May the filthy spot on which your altars stand
be destroyed; may your crops be failures, and your home dilapidated.
May your dead be disturbed in their graves, and may your land become
a feeding place for fishes."

b. Now I make a leaf of Voices—for I have found
    nothing mightier than they are,
And I have found that no word spoken, but
    is beautiful, in its place.
O what is it in me that makes me tremble so
    at voices?
Surely, whoever speaks to me in the right
    voice, him or her I shall follow.
As the water follows the moon, silently
    with fluid steps, anywhere around
    the globe.
All waits for the right voices;
Where is the practis'd and perfect organ? Where
    is the developed soul?
For I see every word utter'd thence has deeper,
    sweeter, new sounds, impossible
    on less terms.
I see brains and lips closed—tympans and temples
    unstruck,
Until that comes which has the quality to strike
    and to unclose,
Until that comes which has the quality to bring
    forth what lies slumbering, forever ready,
    in all words.
        —from Walt Whitman, "Leaves of Grass"

BREATH CONTROL FOR PAUSES AND PHRASES

Before proceeding with exercises for breath control on pauses and phrases,
several factors related to depth and rate of inhalation and control of exhalation should be kept in mind.

1. *Depth of inhalation.* The amount of air, naturally, should be adequate
    to support whatever is spoken on exhalation. Typically, we call words
    spoken on a single inhalation-exhalation cycle a *breath group.* Breath
    groups vary in number of words spoken as well as the manner spoken,
    which has a direct bearing on how much breath is needed for a given
    breath group; for example, the longer the vocal utterance, the greater
    the stress, or the greater the intensity of a given unit, the more air is
    needed per breath group. Even the most demanding sentences should
    require considerably less air than is available to the speaker.

2. *Rate of inhalation.* Inhalation rate depends on several factors, including time pressure, emotion, meaning, and individual differences in structure and capacity. If a speaker is under time pressure to speak quickly, naturally he is going to speed up inhalation. If he is in the middle of a long sentence, he may want to replenish his breath supply. Typically, interphrasal inhalations are shorter than those that initiate a sentence or follow end-stop punctuation (period, semicolon, question mark, etc.), or a significant pause. There is a need to master a technique called *catch breath*, which is used to accomplish various depths of inhalation quickly.

People differ greatly in both the emotion and depth of meaning of what they say, and perhaps even more so in their personality structure. Therefore, breathing techniques must be tailored to the individual. The exercises in this chapter are designed to meet the minimum needs of a wide range of speakers.

Catch Breaths

Catch breaths are used to replenish breath supply quickly when moving from one phrase to another within a sentence. Catch breaths typically occur between phrases within compound or complex sentences. In order to demonstrate a catch breath, have the client visualize the dome-shaped diaphragm at its rest position (e.g., like an inverted bowl). Now picture this muscle in its fully contracted position (i.e., nearly flat). The increase in the volume of the thoracic cavity is great when moving from the dome-shaped rest position to the flat, fully contracted position, and the quicker the movement, the faster air rushes into the lungs. Demonstrate this action by forming an inverted bowl with your hands; lace your fingers lightly and turn your palms down. Now, snap your hands flat with a downward motion. Try to accomplish this in less than half a second.

EXERCISES

In the following exercises, attempt to achieve speed of action of your diaphragm.

1. Observe your clinician as he demonstrates a catch breath. Now, attempt to imitate the movement of his abdominal wall and lateral rib cage as he does this more slowly for you. Attempt to speed up the action.
2. Place the palm of your hand on your abdomen just below the breastbone. On a silent count of one, inhale rapidly. Check the amount of air exhaled by blowing on the back of your hand. Repeat until you have an adequate supply. If you cannot demonstrate success, inhale a little more slowly at first and gradually speed up the action.
3. Place one hand on your abdomen as in Exercise 2 and put the other one in front of your mouth to check the outgoing airstream. Inhale

quickly; now, exhale over a silent count of one to five. Inhale immediately at the end of the silent count and exhale again for another count of five. Repeat this exercise until you demonstrate a satisfactory catch breath.

4. Modify Exercise 3 as follows, always using a silent count. Inhale quickly, exhale over a count of five, then pause, holding your breath without inhaling. Do not close your glottis. Now, exhale over a silent count of five, and immediately after the last count take a catch breath and repeat the exercise. The second step in this exercise, holding the breath with the glottis open, is typical of a pause, and is a maneuver that you will repeat many times while speaking.

5. Now you are ready to add voice to this exercise, provided, of course, that you have mastered the catch breath. The mark, ∨, indicates a catch breath; use it in counting the number chains.
   a. ∨ 1-2-3-4-5 ∨ 1-2-3-4-5 ∨ 1-2-3-4-5 ∨ 1-2-3-4-5
   b. ∨ 1-2-3-4 ∨ 1-2-3-4-5-6-7 ∨ 1-2-3-4-5-6-7-8-9-10-11
   c. ∨ 1-2-3-4-5 ∨ 1-2-3-4-5-6-7-8-9-10-11-12-13-14
   d. ∨ 1-2-3-4-5 ∨ 1-2-3-4-5-6-7-8-9-10-11-12 ∨ 1-2-3-4-5
   e. ∨ 1-2-3-4-5-6-7-8-9-10-11-12-13-14-15 ∨ 1-2-3 ∨ 1-2-3-4-5

6. The mark, /, indicates a pause without taking a breath. Be sure to keep your glottis open during the pause. Pauses need not all be the same length. Perform the following number chains.
   a. ∨ 1-2-3-4-5 / 6-7-8-9-10 ∨ 1-2-3-4-5 / 6-7-8-9-10
   b. ∨ 1-2-3-4-5 / 6-7-8-9-10 ∨ 11-12-13-14-15 / 16-17-18-19-20
   c. ∨ 1-2-3-4-5 / 6-7-8-9-10 / 11-12-13-14-15 ∨ 16-17-18-19-20
   d. ∨ 1-2-3-4 / 5-6-7-8-9-10-11-12 ∨ 13-14-15-16-17-18
   e. ∨ 1-2-3-4-5-6-7-8 / 9-10-11-12 / 13-14-15-16 ∨ 17-18-19-20

7. Practice the number chains below, with // indicating a normal, unhurried inhalation for speech, / indicating pause, and ∨ indicating a catch breath.
   a. // 1-2-3-4-5 ∨ 6-7-8-9-10 // 11-12-13-14-15 ∨ 16-17-18-19-20
   b. // 1-2-3-4-5 / 6-7-8-9-10 // 11-12-13-14-15 / 16-17-18-19-20
   c. // 1-2-3-4-5-6 / 7-8-9 / 10-11-12-13-14 ∨ 15-16-17-18-19-20
   d. // 1-2-3-4-5-6 / 7-8-9-10 // 11-12-13-14-15 / 16-17-18
      ∨ 19-20-21-22
   e. // 1-2-3-4-5-6-7-8 // 9-10-11-12-13-14-15-16 ∨ 17-18-19-20-21

8. Repeat the material in Exercises 5–7, varying pitch patterns and intensity.

Combining Pauses and Phrases and Breath Control

Pauses and phrases are determined by the meaning and emotional content a speaker wishes to communicate and are a highly individualistic matter; therefore, it is not possible to postulate rules governing the use of pauses and phrases. It is possible, however, to state a few guidelines that are useful in developing good breathing habits for meaningful material.

GUIDELINES

1. Pauses and phrases must be tailored to an individual's meaning, emotional content, and capacities.

2. Punctuation in writing can be used as an approximate guide in determining pauses and phrases, particularly the end-stop marks, such as the period, semicolon, question mark, and exclamation mark.

3. Sentences are usually phrased into their most meaningful components. Long sentences should be divided into convenient breath groups.

4. Syntax (word order and grammatical structure) may often be used as a guide to pauses and phrases.

EXERCISE

The following sentences are marked arbitrarily for pauses and phrases. Practice the sentences, using the following marks as guides: // unhurried inhalation for speech; / pause without inhalation; and ∨ catch breath.

a. // The depression led to the fierce and bloody labor-capital wars of the '30s.

b. // He fell over the last hurdle on the turn, / but still won the race handily.

c. // Through all he endured / he maintained his calm / and never lost hope.

d. // Whenever a rancher grew careless, / a band of raiders would swoop down to capture his horses or cattle.

e. // Remember this, Tim Carter, / if you continue to lie, ∨ which I know you are, / *you're as good as dead.*

f. // The young man looked foolish, / and probably felt so, // but there was a resentment in his heart, too, / and a craving for revenge.

g. // She wore skin-tight velvet pants, / and wore them well, // with a white satin blouse, / whose deeply scooped neckline made a mockery of modesty.

h. // The horse and rider came slowly down the hill, / paused a moment, / then continued on, ∨ indicating some measure of indecision on the part of the man in the saddle.

i. // Come fill your cup! // Drink a toast to old Saint Nick!

j. // I'm not leaving you alone, / not for a minute— / not until he's apprehended. ∨ He's dangerous, you know, / already has killed two, ∨ has injured many, / and has left a path of destruction / both in the North / and in the South.

k. ∨ I could not agree with you more! ∨ Now I know the majority were not informed of the truth! ∨ Now I know that the majority were not only not informed of the truth / but were deceived!

l. // From the distance the small dark objects on the ice looked like rocks, / but upon closer inspection, ∨ one could make out the forms of furry animals, / sitting up on their haunches / with their heads buried in their paws.

m. // It was the month of June, / the grass was all white with daisies and the trees with blossoms, ∨ but it was as cold as December.

n. // Put that gun back in its holster! ∨ Move over there by the stove! ∨ All right, Jack, / go get the sheriff.

BREATH CONTROL FOR FORCE

Every speaker should have the ability to regulate the force of his voice, not only for stressing key words, but for increasing or decreasing the over-all intensity of the voice output in relation to phrase and sentence meaning. A change in loudness is directly dependent upon a change in the subglottic breath pressure and involves the muscles of both respiration and phonation.

The exercises that follow are chiefly concerned with the breath control needed for force change. Exercises for projection, stress, and force are included in Chapter 6.

EXERCISES FOR GREATER-THAN-NORMAL BREATH CONTROL

1. Practice exhalation on five distinct puffs. Did you feel your abdominal wall suddenly contract on each one? Repeat until all five puffs are of equal force and duration.

2. Tear off a corner of a piece of paper and place it on a table at least two feet away from your mouth. Can you move it with one puff? Try it again, attempting to gain greater force.

3. Place a piece of 8½ x 11-inch paper just below your lower lip. Direct your breath stream across the surface of the paper. Can you make the paper rise to a nearly horizontal position? Try again.

4. Pretend you are blowing out the candles on a birthday cake on one breath. Now pretend you are attempting to get the smouldering coals of a barbeque going by blowing vigorously on them. Lastly, pretend you have a sticky feather on each fingertip—blow them off, one at a time.

EXERCISES USING MONITORING EQUIPMENT

There are several instruments that can be used to indicate intensity (loudness) levels. Most of them involve some sort of visual indication of the intensity level of the sample spoken.

1. The *VU meter* is used to monitor intensity input of the signal (the voice) into the microphone of a typical public address system. The input signal strength can be raised or lowered by a control dial. Two basic procedures are described below. Use the following sentences for this exercise.

a. How are you today?
b. I don't see him very often.
c. How many times do I have to tell you?
d. Howard and Harvey may not go tomorrow.
e. You never know what the future may bring.

Procedure I

(1) Read the practice sentences above.
(2) Use a quiet conversational voice level, standing four to six inches from the microphone. Keep your intensity and pitch levels relatively constant.
(3) The clinician adjusts the control dial to monitor the vocal input to the meter at 0 (peaks of intensity).
(4) Using the same level of intensity, move back from the microphone until the peaks of intensity drop from 0 to —10.
(5) Without straining, raise your intensity level until the VU meter shows the peaks at 0 again. You have raised your vocal output by 10 dB (decibels).
(6) Using the intensity level achieved in Step 5 above, move back from the microphone until the intensity peaks drop from 0 to —10 dB on the VU meter; now, increase your vocal output until the needle peaks at 0 again on the meter. If successful, you will have increased your output by an additional 10 dB.

Note: An increase from 60 to 70 dB (SPL) is far easier to achieve than raising the level from 70 to 80 dB. It may not be desirable to try a third level, 80 to 90 dB, since vocal strain could easily result.

Procedure II

(1) Use the same sentences as for Procedure I.
(2) Instead of moving back from the microphone, the clinician will turn down the input sensitivity 10 dB as you read. The VU meter should now be made to peak at —10 dB.
(3) Increase your intensity until the instructor signals that you have reached the 0 level on the VU meter.
(4) Steps 2 and 3 can be repeated, which will demand that you increase your vocal output 10 dB to reach 0 once more.

2. Any sound level meter can be used to indicate intensity level of vocal output and is perhaps even simpler to handle then the VU meter in the two procedures presented above. The portable types of sound-level meters can be very useful and are easily handled.[1]

Procedure

(1) Place the sound-level meter at a convenient place where it can be read easily, such as a table.

(2) Using the sentences in Exercise 1 above, establish your base output level, using a quiet, conversational voice. The clinician will adjust the sound-level meter until he obtains a reading.

(3) Repeat the reading, using a slightly greater intensity level (one consistent with more animated conversation). The clinician adjusts the sound level meter and obtains a reading. If you have not increased your intensity enough, your clinician may signal you to increase your vocal output. The clinician sets the level to be achieved in this step.

(4) The clinician may manipulate the intensity of the client's vocal output over a wide range. Likewise, the client can be instructed to adjust the dials for measuring all levels for himself and can practice different kinds of materials, provided he is able to stay within the objectives of the exercise.

3. Using the same equipment as in Exercises 1 or 2 above, project your voice to imaginary listeners under several experimental conditions: (a) to one other person at close range, (b) to three persons seated in a quiet living room, and (c) to fifteen persons seated around a table in a noisy restaurant. Avoid tension and be careful not to strain your voice. Depend on intensity rather than raising your basic pitch level for projection. Repeat, paying particular attention to the proprioceptive-tactile-kinesthetic sensations for each level. The ability to monitor intensity by PTK is extremely important and should be mastered at this stage of training.

EXERCISES FOR VARYING LEVELS OF FORCE

1. Practice the following words, using three levels of force: quiet, normal, and loud conversational levels. Pay particular attention to control of breathing. Do not raise pitch, avoid tension, and prolong the words slightly. To reduce tension, keep the tone quality on the breathy side.

yes	roll	now	my	loam
hold	ho	boy	may	lamb
high	one	fall	moan	law

2. Practice the following sentences, using three levels of force (quiet, normal, and loud). Avoid tension and try to rely chiefly upon breath pressure to accomplish your goal.

---

[1] The General Radio sound-level meter (Model 1551c) and the portable Bruel and Kjaer sound-level meter (Model 2203) are both ideal for this kind of work.

   a. Halt! Who goes there?

   b. Where are you going?

   c. Release your tensions by progressive relaxation.

   d. Our rugged land stretched down to the water's edge.

   e. Roll on, thou deep and dark blue ocean, roll!

   f. How many volunteers have been called?

   g. Walter, I want you to come home this minute!

   h. Rouse yourselves from your listless indolence and rebel!

   i. I call upon all of you to support me tomorrow night!

   j. How high does the mountain tower over the valley?

3. Practice the three short selections that follow, using the instructions in Exercises 1 and 2 above.

   a. God of our fathers, known of old,
       Lord of our far-flung battle-line,
    Beneath whose awful Hand we hold
       Dominion over palm and pine—
    Lord God of Hosts, be with us yet,
    Lest we forget—lest we forget!

    The tumult and the shouting dies;
       The Captains and the Kings depart:
    Still stands Thine ancient sacrifice,
       An humble and a contrite heart.
    Lord God of Hosts, be with us yet,
    Lest we forget—lest we forget!
       —from Rudyard Kipling, "Recessional"

   b. A dispute once arose between the Wind and the Sun, which was the stronger of the two, and they agreed to put the point upon this issue, that whichever soonest made a traveller take off his cloak, should be accounted the more powerful. The Wind began, and blew with all his might and main a blast, cold and fierce as a Thracian storm; but the stronger he blew the closer the traveller wrapped his cloak around him, and the tighter he grasped it with his hands. Then broke out the Sun: with his welcome beams he dispersed the vapour and the cold; the traveller felt the genial warmth, and as the Sun shone brighter and brighter, he sat down, overcome with the heat, and cast his cloak on the ground.
       —from Aesop, "The Wind and the Sun"

   c. I SHOT an arrow into the air,
    It fell to earth, I knew not where;
    For, so swiftly it flew, the sight
    Could not follow it in its flight.
    I breathed a song into the air,

It fell to earth, I knew not where;
For who has sight so keen and strong
That it can follow the flight of song?
Long, long afterward, in an oak
I found the arrow, still unbroke;
And the song, from beginning to end,
I found again in the heart of a friend.
　　　—Henry Wadsworth Longfellow,
　　　"The Arrow and The Song"

SELECTIONS FOR PRACTICE

1. Break, break, break,
　　　On thy cold gray stones, O Sea!
　　And I would that my tongue could utter
　　　The thoughts that arise in me.

　　O, well for the fisherman's boy,
　　　That he shouts with his sister at play!
　　O, well for the sailor lad,
　　　That he sings in his boat on the bay!

　　And the stately ships go on
　　　To their haven under the hill;
　　But O for the touch of a vanish'd hand,
　　　And the sound of a voice that is still!

　　Break, break, break,
　　　At the foot of thy crags, O Sea!
　　But the tender grace of a day that is dead
　　　Will never come back to me.
　　　　　—Alfred Lord Tennyson, "Break, Break, Break"

2.　　Unfathomable Sea! whose waves are years,
　　　　Ocean of Time, whose waters of deep woe
　　　Are brackish with the salt of human tears!
　　　　Thou shoreless flood, which in thy ebb
　　　　　and flow
　　　Clapest the limits of mortality,
　　　And sick of prey, yet howling on for more,
　Vomitest thy wrecks on its inhospitable shore;
　　　Treacherous in calm, and terrible in storm,
　　　　　Who shall put forth on thee,
　　　　　Unfathomable Sea?
　　　　　　—Percy Bysshe Shelley, "Time"

3. The full streams feed on flower of rushes,
　　　Ripe grasses trammel a traveling foot,

The faint fresh flame of the young year flushes
    From leaf to flower and flower to fruit;
        —from Algernon Charles Swinburne, "Atalanta in Calydon"

4. No stir in the air, no stir in the sea,
The ship was still as she could be;
Her sails from heaven received no motion;
Her keel was steady in the ocean.
        —from Robert Southey, "The Inchcape Rock"

5. This has been the season of thickening clouds, hailstorms,
shattering thunder, fireworks in the sky, cloudbursts,
swollen streams—and finally that which all feared—massive
floods.

6. A slumber did my spirit seal;
I had no human fears;
She seemed a thing that could not feel
The touch of earthy years.

No motion has she now, no force;
She neither hears nor sees;
Rolled round in earth's diurnal course,
With rocks, and stones, and trees.
        —from William Wordsworth, "Lucy"

7. Adapt yourself to change as the willow tree adapts itself to the weather. When the harsh winds of circumstance sweep across the landscape of your life, bow gracefully, bend gently, adapt graciously.

You are wise to study well the ways of the willow. In the face of change, in the throes of adversity, in the midst of conflict and crisis, the willow willingly bends its branches but refuses to release its roots.

Silently, serenely, securely, sink your own roots into the depths of a dependable faith. Then, like the willow, you can confidently confront and courageously conquer the challenge of change.
        —anon.

8. But it is useless to try to try to describe the Grand Canyon. Those who have not seen it will not believe any possible description; and those who have seen it know that it cannot be painted in either pigments or words.

I have heard rumors of visitors who were disappointed. The same people will be disappointed at the Day of Judgment. In fact, the Grand Canyon is a sort of landscape Day of Judgment. It is not a show place, a beauty spot, but a revelation. The Colorado River, which is powerful, turbulent, and so thick with silt that it is like a saw, made it with the help of the erosive forces of rain, frost, and wind, and some strange geological accidents; and all these together have been hard at work on it for the last seven or eight million years. It is the largest of the eighteen canyons of the Colorado River, is over two hundred miles long, has an average width of twelve miles, and is a good mile deep. It is the world's supreme example of erosion. But this is not what it really is. It is, I repeat, a revelation. The Colorado River made it, but you feel when you are there that God gave the Colorado River its instructions. It is all Beethoven's nine symphonies in stone and magic light. Even to remember that it is still there lifts up the heart. If I were an American, I should make my remembrance of it the final test of men, art, and policies. I should ask myself: Is this good enough to exist in the same country as the Canyon? How would I feel about this man, this kind of art, these political measures, if I were near that Rim? Every member or officer of the Federal Government ought to remind himself, with triumphant pride, that he is on the staff of the Grand Canyon.

—from J. B. Priestley, "Midnight in the Desert"

9. All things are double, one against another.—Tit for tat; an eye for an eye; a tooth for a tooth; blood for blood; measure for measure; love for love.—Give, and it shall be given you.—He that watereth shall be watered himself.—What will you have? quoth God; pay for it and take it.—Nothing venture, nothing have.—Thou shalt be paid exactly for what thou hast done, no more, no less.—Who doth not work shall not eat.—Harm watch, harm catch.—Curses always recoil on the head of him who imprecates them.—If you put a chain around the neck of a slave, the other end fastens itself around your own.—Bad counsel confounds the adviser.—The Devil is an ass.

It is thus written, because it is thus in life. Our action is overmastered and characterized above our will by the law of nature. We aim at a petty end quite aside from the public good, but our act arranges itself by irresistible magnetism in a line with the poles of the world.

—from Ralph Waldo Emerson, "Compensation"

9

Phonation

Modifying phonatory behavior is concerned primarily with two basic approaches: (a) modifying the hypovalved larynx and associated vibrator behaviors and (b) modifying the hypervalved larynx and associated vibrator behaviors. The degree of valving may not relate to the mode of oscillation of the vocal folds; therefore, the assessment should clarify the relationship of both valving and oscillation behavior to the problem. In modifying the *hypovalved* larynx, the clinician attempts to have the client use the contrast behavior of *hypervalving*. In changing the behavior of the *hypervalved* larynx, the contrast behavior of *hypovalving* is used (see Chapter 4).

The concept of the continuum of valving, presented in Figure 1.1, is useful in explaining to the client the type of valving behavior that is desired. In modifying the behavior of the client with a hypervalved larynx, the contrast behavior of hypovalving is used to separate the vocal folds during vibration, eliminate struggle behaviors, insure greater airflow, and induce a more relaxed approach to phonation. Under these conditions of phonation, the mode of oscillation will not be as restricted or impaired as with more extreme forms of hypervalving. After easy, effortless hypovalved phonation is established and stabilized, phonation is then shaped toward optimal laryngeal behaviors. In modifying the laryngeal behavior of the client with a voice problem of hypovalving, the contrast behavior of hypervalving is used to insure closer approximation of the vocal folds, more efficient utilization of the airflow, and unhampered vocal fold vibration. In both approaches, then, the clinician uses an *overcompensation* of valving behavior, and, if successful, shapes phonation toward optimal production.

Contrasting behaviors are used throughout the training program and not limited to valving alone; the clinician may use contrasts of low- versus high-fundamental frequency, low- versus high-intensity levels, or short versus long duration of syllables. Indeed, the use of contrasting behaviors should be part of every aspect of a behavior modification program for voice.

INITIATING PHONATION

The Use of Hypervalving

Hypervalving is used as the compensatory, contrasting approach to voice disorders associated with hypovalving. The presentation in Chapter 4 should be reviewed before beginning these procedures. This type of approach utilizes the initiation of phonation from the fully adducted position of the vocal folds. The *degree of tightness* of closure may be varied, depending on the needs of the client. The terms glottal shock, glottal attack, hard attack, glottal plosive, and coup de glotte are all used to indicate the fully adducted approach to the initiation of phonation. Since these terms cannot be used to describe a continuum of tight closures (i.e., from tight to very tight), the clinician will need to explain to the client the degree of closure he wants. In this text, the term glottal shock will be used to indicate slightly less tightness of closure than coup de glotte.

PROCEDURES

1. *Coup de glotte.* The vocal folds are adducted and held firmly pressed together to permit a high degree of subglottic breath pressure increase; the pressure is suddenly released into a vocal tone. The arms may be used to good advantage to augment the moment of release by (a) bending the arms at the elbows, (b) holding the arms laterally at about neck level, (c) clenching the fists tightly, and (d) suddenly lashing downward with the arms as the air pressure is released into a grunt or any other vocalization desired by the clinician (e.g., [ɑ], [oʊ], *I, out*).

   Coup de glotte can be used in a pushing-release activity. Have the client push strenuously against a desk while impounding and increasing breath pressure at the glottis; then, have him release his breath suddenly, as described above.

2. *Glottal shock.* The term glottal shock has been used to describe the onset of voice from the fully adducted position of the vocal folds. Glottal shock occurs in most voices when the speaker attempts to stress a word beginning with a vowel (e.g., *aim, any*). Glottal shock may be described as follows: (a) the vocal folds are adducted and held under tension while subglottic breath pressure increases, (b) the airflow is impounded, (c) the air is released explosively, and (d) an audible "click" or glottal plosive is heard as sound is initiated. Because of the hypervalving of the larynx and tension in the pharynx, the vowel following the glottal shock is often strident in quality. The intensity of the glottal shock depends on the degree of implosion and explosion of the air. While glottal shock is not desirable in optimal speech production,

it is useful in hypervalving the larynx of a person with a hypovalving voice problem. The four exercises below are typical of those used for a glottal shock approach to phonation.

3. *The use of humming.* Humming can be very useful in establishing good approximation of the vocal folds. The resistance to the airflow is slightly greater through the pharyngo-nasal air route than in the pharyngo-oral route and may account for the more fortunate adjustment of the vocal folds while humming. Have the client hum lightly at his optimum pitch level. Use a monotone before attempting inflections of the tone. Work on the hypovalved side of the continuum during early attempts at voice production. Later, move toward optimal valving. Concentrate upon focusing the tone with easy, low intensity vocal attempts. Let the airflow rush through the glottal chink, as in [h], then initiate the hum. Repeat several times, then move to low vowels, for example, [ɑ], [aʊ], and [ɔ].

EXERCISES

1. Perform the following words in two ways, first with a glottal shock, then without it. Attempt to retain the voice quality achieved on the first utterance.

I	act	ate	ore	are
idle	apt	aim	omen	arm
idea	ample	able	order	arbor
ire	adder	air	orchid	argue
item	ask	age	ordeal	alter

2. Perform each of the word pairs below as follows: (a) use a glottal shock to initiate the first word and (b) try to maintain the same voice quality achieved on the vowel in the pair on the second word.

eve-heave	arm-harm	air-hair	arbor-harbor	are-heart
ore-hoar	eye-high	eat-heat	am-ham	old-hold
odd-hod	eel-heel	ail-hail	it-hit	itch-hitch
else-health	ohm-home	and-hand	act-hacked	oh-ho
at-hat	empty-hemp	ill-hill	ought-hot	owe-hotel

3. Perform the following pairs of words, using a glottal shock to initiate the first word but not the second. Try to maintain the same voice quality on the second vowel as on the first.

each-each	arm-arm	able-able	item-item	etch-etch
every-every	act-act	air-air	amber-amber	ouch-ouch
any-any	only-only	even-even	age-age	aid-aid
out-out	undue-undue	eighty-eighty	odor-odor	add-add
and-and	odd-odd	anti-anti	order-order	into-into

4. Use a glottal shock on all words beginning with vowels in the sentences below. When you have achieved a high level of success, attempt to perform the sentences without the glottal attack, but try to maintain the same voice quality attained on the glottal shock approach.

a. It's odd that Alice is not at Eileen's tea.
b. Each and every one of us ought to be aware of it.
c. Any ape is apt to ape an actor.
d. Ada aided Ellen and Edward in anchoring the skiff.
e. Aim! Aim! Aram yelled, as he waved his arms aimlessly.

The Use of Hypovalving

The contrasting behavior of hypovalving is used in initiating phonation for voice disorders associated with hypervalving. The presentation in Chapter 4 should be reviewed before working with this type of problem.

PROCEDURES

1. *The aspirate attack.* This approach to initiating voice production uses the same principles as for Procedure 3 below but typically applies only to breathy and extremely breathy qualities in initiating syllables (e.g., *ha, he, hey, he, own, know*). A generous amount of airflow and control of the breathy voice quality characterize this method of initiating tone.
2. *Yawn-phonation.* The yawn induces relaxation in both the pharynx and larynx and prepares the client for easy phonation. The yawn stretches laryngeal and pharyngeal muscles. Have the client yawn, then have him release airflow during the yawn and phonate a breathy [ɑ]. The yawn may be used as a way to teaching the client to feel the difference between tension and relaxation in phonation.
3. *Modifying airflow.* Since clients who hypervalve their larynxes generally do not use an adequate flow of air during phonation, increasing airflow while hypovalving the vocal folds will help to modify the behavior. It may be necessary to work on increasing breath supply and control first before combining airflow and phonation drills. Have the client use ample airflow on exhalation under several degrees of hypovalving:
    (a) Vocal folds completely abducted; very little turbulence.
    (b) Vocal folds in whisper position; turbulence, but no oscillation of folds (no phonation).
    (c) Vocal folds approximated lightly; vocal folds vibrating minimally; phonation very breathy.
    (d) Nearly full fold vibration of vocal folds, but with breathy quality.
    Monitor the airflow by placing your hand in front of the client's mouth. Insist on a generous flow of air. Have the client monitor his own airflow by the same method. Experiment with each of the degrees of closure described above until the client can do them easily on demand.

SUSTAINED PHONATION

The first phase of either approach to modifying laryngeal behaviors is chiefly concerned with initiating the tone. After this step has been accomplished, consideration must be given to sustaining phonation over time.

Several procedures may be used, including (a) decreasing on-off phonation, (b) tonal and singing approaches to sustained phonation, and (c) using the breathy and yawn-sigh approaches to sustained hypovalving.

Decreasing On-Off Phonation

In the optimal use of voice, speakers usually utter a series of phonemes in a continuous chain within phrases and breath groups. Many clients with voice problems tend to use more on-off phonation than is necessary, particularly those who exhibit struggle behavior. If a client has a tendency to use off phonation after completing words within phrases, a choppy, uneven delivery is apparent, and the flow of syllables is unnecessarily interrupted. Several exercises for increasing phonation by decreasing off phonation between words are given below.

EXERCISES

1. Perform the following phrases in two ways: (a) Say each word individually and do not use linking, noting the "choppy" delivery; and (b) join the syllables together in one continuous flow. Practice the latter approach until the utterance is smooth and contains good emphasis of stressed syllables within the chain.
   a. go tomorrow
      go tomorrow morning
      will go tomorrow morning
      Harry will go tomorrow morning.
   b. soon
      home soon
      will come home soon
      ought to come home soon
      He ought to come home soon.
   c. the spring
      nests in the spring
      build their nests in the spring
      Robins build their nests in the spring.
   d. ocean
      blue ocean
      deep and dark blue ocean
      Roll on, thou deep and dark blue ocean, Roll!
2. Intrusive consonants often appear between syllables when the last phoneme of the first word and the first phoneme of the second word favor the development of a glide. Perform the following words in several ways: (a) with on-off phonation between words; (b) with linking, but without an intrusive glide; and (c) with a strong intrusive glide.

[r]	[w]	[j]
here are	do it	he undertakes
mother or	how is	high every
pier is	who am	my only
fair art	amino acids	try any

3. Through linking and stress, final consonants often become the first phoneme in the syllables that follow them. Practice the following words without linking, then with linking and stress.

fall out	hum up	can open
fill in	then agree	con artist
feel only	thumb only	Allen agrees
Bill indicates	problem opens	common opinion

4. Additional materials for practice may be found in the section on sustained resonance, pp. 169–170.

The Tonal Approach

PROCEDURES

Have the client practice all steps in the following procedure. Do not go on to a succeeding step until the one under consideration has been accomplished successfully.

1. Hum a tone that is at the client's optimum pitch level.[1] If the clinician has difficulty in modeling the tone adequately because of a major difference in voice type (e.g., male-female, bass-tenor), a recorded model may be used. Have the client produce a similar tone. Several attempts may be necessary to adjust the client's vocal output.[2] A light, slightly breathy tone is desirable. Be sure that the client uses plenty of airflow during tone production. Use a monopitch and hold the tone steady (without vibrato or tremulo).

2. While humming with the lips lightly closed, form the vowel [i] and open your mouth. The clinician should model the tone first, then the client should attempt to echo it. Adjust the client's tone by explaining and modeling. Continue until the tone is satisfactory. Keep the intensity of the tone at a low level, but with enough force to sustain the voice without a pitch break.

3. Use the same procedure as in Step 2, then merge slowly from [i] to [u] and finally to [ɑ]. The clinician should model the tone, then listen critically to the response of the client. Use specific instructions, such as "A little more breathy," "Use more airflow," "A little less force," or "Listen closely to me and try to imitate my voice." Several repeti-

[1] The concept of optimum pitch is helpful here. Locate the optimum pitch of the client (for procedure, see Chapter 6). If the client has difficulty in establishing an optimum level, the clinician should select a pitch level that is the most comfortable and easy for him.
[2] If the client is unable to follow directions on Steps 1–3 of this procedure because of difficulty in humming or intoning, skip to Step 4.

tions are usually necessary to shape the client's tone to a satisfactory result.

4. Intone an easy, somewhat breathy [ɑ] sound using a monopitch. Repeat several times, attempting to improve upon the quality of the sound.

5. Repeat the syllable [ɑ] in an easy, effortless way, prolonging both the [h] and [ɑ], again using a monopitch. Modeling of the quality wanted as well as explanation of what to do should be used liberally by the clinician at this point. Do not be in a hurry to move on to the next step.

6. Repeat Step 5, only this time add a falling inflection to the tone. Diminish the tone to extinction by relaxing the vocal folds selectively. Continue modeling the tone and having the client repeat it until the vocal output is satisfactory.

7. Repeat Step 5, only this time use a rising inflection. Diminish the voice to extinction. The tone should blend smoothly into a falsetto in the upward glide. Many persons are unable to glide smoothly, as the upward glide involves added tension if loudness is not decreased; practice is usually required before this maneuver can be done satisfactorily.[3] Ability to diminish the vocal tone in upward inflections is a most desirable maneuver for the client to master, since this type of glide is quite common in speech.

8. Repeat Steps 1 through 7, using *aw* [ɔ] instead of *ah* [ɑ].

9. Repeat Steps 1 through 7, using *oh* [oʊ] instead of *aw* [ɔ].
   Note: Steps 8 and 9 may be used optionally, or as a variation in daily drill.

10. Have the client demonstrate his ability to move successfully from Step 1 through 7 without prompting. Assign these steps to be practiced three times a day.

11. After the client has achieved a satisfactory level of performance on Steps 1–10, move on to the Core Materials in the last section of this chapter. It may be necessary, from time to time, to come back to working with vowels and diphthongs in order to reestablish the voice quality desired, particularly as the meaningful material becomes more difficult.

12. Perform the procedure for adjusting and stabilizing the voice, pp. 156–157.

The Singing Approach

Singing requires sustained phonation within breath groups and may be used as a method of voice training. The rationale, requirements, guidelines, and procedures for the singing approach are presented in Chapter 11.

---

[3] If difficulty is encountered in any of the steps, it is often wise for the client to avoid hypervalving by using a little more breathiness.

SUSTAINED HYPOVALVING

The Breathy Approach

Many voice specialists have relied exclusively upon utilizing breathy initiation of tone and breathy speech as their entire approach to voice rehabilitation for clients who hypervalve their larynxes. The principle underlying this type of approach is that the client uses too tight closure of the vocal folds on phonation and is not only producing an inappropriate voice quality, but is subjecting his laryngeal structures to trauma and possible damage.

Relaxation and breathing exercises can be incorporated into the breathy approach without difficulty. It may not be necessary to follow all of the steps in the procedure below, as the client may make rapid progress; therefore, the stabilization and carry-over phases of training can be speeded up.

PROCEDURES

1. Explain to the client that his way of producing voice involves excess tension and force and that a new adjustment of the valving mechanism is needed. Demonstrate the difference between hypervalving and hypovalving, modeling each.
2. Present a program of auditory discrimination of hypovalved, optimally produced, and hypervalved items.
3. Demonstrate the level of breathiness desired on the word *high*. Have the client echo your models, making adjustments if the responses are too breathy or too tense. Regulate the amount of airflow the client uses by having him match your model. Several other words may be used, such as *how, hey, ha, hoe, way, my, know*. Use a downward inflection, optimum pitch level, and low levels of intensity on all attempts.
4. Progress to two-word, meaningful phrases, such as *how high, my name, I know*. Make the same adjustments as in Step 3. Turn to the Core Materials near the end of this chapter and complete Programs I–III, using the same breathy approach on all samples. Work for ease in production, with breathy tone quality, downward inflections on the word or phrase endings, and low levels of intensity.
5. After the client has gained control of his new voice, continue with the Core Materials and complete the remainder of the programs, IV–VIII. Try to fade some of the client's breathiness and shape vocal output toward more tonality, but be sure to remain on the breathy side of optimal production.
6. Stabilize the new voice in carry-over drills. Encourage the client to use his "new voice" as much as possible. Check on his ability to self-monitor his speech.
7. Perform the procedure for stabilizing and adjusting the voice, pp. 156–157.

The Yawn-Sigh Approach

Combining yawning and phonation has been a routine approach to voice problems for decades. The approach is based upon the following principles: (a) Yawning is nature's method of relaxing the mouth, throat, and larynx; (b) yawning for the most part usually involves a substantial air intake (not always, but usually) and generally continues on through exhalation; and (c) initiation of tone during and after the yawn utilizes naturally induced relaxation, a good breath supply, and an acceptable preparatory set for vocalization. Like the breathy approach, this method of voice training is effective in treating persons with hypervalved larynxes and hypertense muscles throughout the speech mechanism.

PROCEDURES

1. Discuss yawning with the client and ask him if he can yawn readily. Present various types of yawning, ranging from the small, half-stifled yawn of the bored auditor to the full, open-mouthed variety so often seen in drowsy college students.
2. Demonstrate the type of yawn needed for training—open-mouthed; substantial air intake; full stretch of the soft palate and pharyngeal walls; and a gentle release of the airstream. It is necessary to start with a fully developed yawn that can be faded toward a less extensive one as the program progresses. Have the client try a similar type of yawn and do not go on until he has done this step to your satisfaction. The client may have to get into the mood for this type of maneuver. Most people can yawn nicely after getting over their inhibitions.
3. During the exhalation phase of the yawn cycle, ask the patient to sigh *ah* [ɑ]. Model what you want if the *ah* is done improperly. Use plenty of airflow on exhalation to encourage breathiness.
4. After the sigh has been produced satisfactorily, shape the *ah* sound into a shorter syllable, fading the more obvious outward manifestations of the yawn (i.e., eyes closing, mouth stretched beyond the normal range for speech, etc.). Use optimum pitch, downward inflections, and prolonged duration.
5. Introduce self-monitoring of how the yawn *feels* while sighing *ah*. Up to this point, you have been primarily concerned with affecting a yawn, getting a good release of air, and developing a good breathy sign [ɑ], which is done by monitoring the acoustic output along with visual appearance of the yawn. Several trials concentrating upon the proprio-ceptive-tactile-kinesthetic involvement of the process are needed to complete this step. Be particularly aware of the *feel* of this process at the onset of tone. *You will be referring back to this step throughout the training sequence.*
6. Do Steps 3 and 4, using various low vowels and diphthongs. The sounds, *aw, oh, I,* and *ow* ([ɔ], [oʊ], [aɪ], and [aʊ]), are suggested.

7. The client must now learn to monitor *good, fair,* and *poor* productions consistently. A program of discrimination training, using the Language Master or loop tape recorder, is probably the best way to accomplish this step. If arranged programmatically, work for 80 percent of all productions being judged correctly.

8. The client must now be taught how to carry over the good results of yawn-sigh into meaningful speech.[4] It is best that this process be done systematically, moving from easy to difficult materials. Therefore, perform all the Core Material programs, using the yawn-sigh approach.

9. After completing the Core Materials, perform the voice stabilizing and adjusting procedure that follows.

ADJUSTING AND STABILIZING THE VOICE

Very often the quality of the client's voice will be "satisfactory" but little more, after completing a program of training utilizing any of the above approaches to sustaining phonation. As a terminal phase of training, it may be wise to develop flexibility and strength in the client's voice over a range of voice qualities. Five levels of adjustment are recommended for this type of training:

Level I: Whisper; no vocal fold oscillation
Level II: Less breathy than Level I; minimal fold vibration
Level III: Slightly breathy; less than optimal voice quality
Level IV: Optimal quality; no breathiness, easy production
Level V: Strident quality; hypervalved larynx; no noise components, however

PROCEDURES

1. Model the five levels for the client, using the word list on p. 159. The client should be able to identify all levels of adjustment when they are presented randomly. Continue the discrimination program until the client has achieved a high level of success.

2. Model Level I for the client and have him echo the quality presented. When Level I is established, go on to Level II; shape the client's response until it matches the modeled stimulus. Continue with Levels III and IV in the same manner. Be sure the client can produce each level correctly. Using Level V is optional. If Level V is difficult to produce, it may be eliminated from the procedure. Use the materials in Programs I–III of the Core Materials for Step 2.

---

[4] At any time during the training with meaningful speech, it is often advisable to return to Steps 1–6 of the yawn-sigh approach, particularly if the client uses inappropriate vocal behavior consistently.

3. Model the four levels randomly and have the client attempt to produce each of these accurately. Use the Language Master or a loop tape recorder to train the client to make correct responses and judgments. Work toward more stringent criteria of success as the client begins to achieve a higher level of correct responses.
4. After the client has demonstrated the ability to produce four distinct voice qualities (Levels I–IV), continue with Programs IV–VIII of the Core Materials, working for stabilization of Levels III and IV with successively more difficult material. The terminal goal should be consistent use of Level IV voice quality, with the ability to move to Level III or even II, when needed.

The ability to hypovalve the larynx at will can be a valuable asset for the client who consistently hypervalves. Recommend that he use Level III occasionally in everyday life, particularly if he is forced to talk extensively or if fatigue and tension emerge.

CORE MATERIALS

The core materials presented in this section are arranged in columns of frames to permit maximum flexibility in their use. The clinician may elect to present the syllables, words, phrases, or sentences independently, varying and improvising his correctional techniques to suit his client's needs. The arrangement is also ideally suited for using an operant conditioning approach to training, which can be done programmatically, if desired.

Program I
Voiceless Fricative and Vowel

Frames	Frames	Frames	Frames	Frames
1 ha	11 how	21 hoe	31 who	41 how
2 haw	12 high	22 haw	32 hay	42 hoy
3 hay	13 haw	23 how	33 hoe	43 who
4 high	14 who	24 ha	34 high	44 high
5 hoy	15 he	25 hoy	35 haw	45 he
6 how	16 ha	26 he	36 hoy	46 hay
7 hoe	17 hay	27 hay	37 ha	47 high
8 who	18 hoy	28 ha	38 how	48 ha
9 he	19 hoe	29 high	39 hoe	49 haw
10 haw	20 high	30 haw	40 hay	50 who

Program II
Vowel-Consonant

Frames	Frames	Frames	Frames	Frames
1 arm	11 ode	21 earn	31 earn	41 out
2 arch	12 own	22 earl	32 alm	42 ark
3 alm	13 our	23 urge	33 art	43 owe
4 are	14 out	24 odd	34 ounce	44 awe
5 art	15 owe	25 on	35 I'm	45 ounce
6 ark	16 ounce	26 are	36 own	46 earn
7 all	17 ice	27 all	37 ought	47 all
8 awe	18 I'm	28 ohm	38 ode	48 alm
9 ought	19 isle	29 our	39 arch	49 ohm
10 ohm	20 up	30 ice	40 up	50 isle

Program III
Consonant-Vowel

Frames	Frames	Frames	Frames	Frames
1 rah	11 no	21 nigh	31 nay	41 row
2 raw	12 woe	22 now	32 raw	42 low
3 row	13 ray	23 way	33 low	43 no
4 la	14 rye	24 wow	34 mow	44 rye
5 law	15 row	25 rah	35 woe	45 lie
6 low	16 lay	26 la	36 rye	46 way
7 ma	17 lie	27 ma	37 lie	47 la
8 maw	18 may	28 gnaw	38 nigh	48 lay
9 mow	19 my	29 ray	39 wow	49 woe
10 gnaw	20 nay	30 lay	40 ma	50 my

Program IV
Consonant-Vowel-Consonant

Frames	Frames	Frames	Frames	Frames
1 role	11 mine	21 warn	31 shown	41 loan
2 mole	12 moan	22 wire	32 shared	42 lime
3 rile	13 lone	23 morn	33 shawl	43 wash
4 wile	14 line	24 mired	34 shame	44 loam
5 wail	15 loll	25 wiles	35 shires	45 nail
6 male	16 lawn	26 mares	36 shores	46 nor
7 maim	17 wall	27 wrong	37 rile	47 gnome
8 mile	18 wan	28 long	38 rale	48 moan
9 mall	19 worn	29 shales	39 roan	49 rhyme
10 main	20 lane	30 shine	40 rime	50 rain

Program V
Disyllabic Words

Frames	Frames	Frames	Frames
1 mushroom	14 houseboy	27 shakedown	39 daylight
2 farewell	15 boardwalk	28 sunset	40 outweigh
3 daybreak	16 boneyard	29 northwest	41 drawbridge
4 oatmeal	17 limelight	30 nightmare	42 baseball
5 inkwell	18 whiplash	31 toothbrush	43 armchair
6 hotdog	19 shoreline	32 doormat	44 horseshoe
7 railroad	20 barnyard	33 iceberg	45 nightcap
8 cowboy	21 hardware	34 eardrum	46 forlorn
9 playmate	22 highboy	35 headlight	47 forewarn
10 mailman	23 highbrow	36 hothouse	48 woodwork
11 cupcake	24 wireworm	37 birthday	49 rainbow
12 workshop	25 shortcake	38 airplane	50 stagecoach
13 lighthouse	26 duckpond		

Program VI
Phrases

Frames	Frames	Frames	Frames	Frames
1 in the house	11 down the hill	21 to the man	31 of the rain	41 on the moon
2 of the car	12 up a bit	22 for a boy	32 of the wash	42 to a star
3 in a minute	13 down a little	23 in the box	33 on the shore	43 of a fish
4 of a mile	14 on the level	24 in the book	34 to the cow	44 in a hurry
5 by the sea	15 on the truck	25 on the lawn	35 of a coach	45 from the lighthouse
6 from the room	16 for the same	26 to the mall	36 to the end	46 to the station
7 to the train	17 for a law	27 in the main	37 by the way	47 of the same
8 around the block	18 to an aunt	28 to the mole	38 on the road	48 in a hurry
9 around the ship	19 for the best	29 of the lime	39 to a horse	49 of a hothouse
10 up the ladder	20 on a lot	30 by the nail	40 on the loam	50 to the sunshine

Program VII
Developmental Sentences

Frames	Frames	Frames
1 love	17 lamb	33 house
2 in love	18 the lamb	34 the house
3 fell in love	19 eyed the lamb	35 struck the house
4 She fell in love.	20 The lion eyed the lamb.	36 Lightning struck the house.
5 well	21 morning	37 lunch
6 him well	22 in the morning	38 his lunch
7 know him well	23 early in the morning	39 ate his lunch
8 I know him well.	24 Rise early in the morning.	40 Howard ate his lunch.
9 horse	25 ground	41 star
10 the horse	26 to the ground	42 the star
11 roped the horse	27 fell to the ground	43 saw the star
12 The cowboy roped the horse.	28 The ball fell to the ground.	44 The astronomer saw the star.
13 barnyard	29 down	45 boy
14 in the barnyard	30 sign down	46 funny boy
15 played in the barnyard	31 blew the sign down	47 at the funny boy
16 George played in the barnyard.	32 The wind blew the sign down.	48 She laughed at the funny boy.

Program VIII
Sentences

1. Shadrach, Meshach, and Abednego came out from the fiery furnace.
2. The renowned rajah waited in the downpour for the mailman to bring the mysterious package.
3. To the wily wireworm the lima bean is like a cupcake.
4. While roaming the range at nightfall, the cowboy found the old boneyard.
5. As the fog began to lift, the old lighthouse emerged high on a promontory above the jagged shoreline.
6. While grandpa drank his usual nightcap, grandma ate her shortcake.

Program VIII (continued)
Sentences

7. The role of the crafty clown was played by a famous Broadway actor.
8. The module was designed to fit even the most demanding architectural plan.
9. Chang, our erstwhile houseboy, was shanghaied after the shakedown, and awoke from the nightmare in Bombay.
10. The hardware on the highboy was easy to maintain.

SELECTIONS FOR PRACTICE

1. Sweet and low, sweet and low,
      Wind of the western sea,
   Low, low, breathe and blow,
      Wind of the western sea!
   Over the rolling waters go,
   Come from the dying moon, and blow,
      Blow him again to me;
   While my little one, while my pretty one, sleeps.

   Sleep and rest, sleep and rest,
      Father will come to thee soon;
   Rest, rest, on mother's breast,
      Father will come to thee soon;
   Father will come to his babe in the nest
   Silver sails all out of the west
      Under the silver moon;
   Sleep, my little one, sleep, my pretty one, sleep.
                    —Alfred Lord Tennyson, "Sweet and Low"

2. I wandered lonely as a cloud
   That floats on high o'er vales and hills,
   When all at once I saw a crowd,
   A host, of golden daffodils,
   Beside the lake, beneath the trees,
   Fluttering and dancing in the breeze.

   Continuous as the stars that shine
   And twinkle on the milky way,
   They stretched in never-ending line
   Along the margin of a bay:
   Ten thousand saw I at a glance,
   Tossing their heads in sprightly dance.

   The waves beside them danced, but they
   Outdid the sparkling waves in glee—

A poet could not but be gay
In such a jocund company.
I gazed—and gazed—but little thought
What wealth the show to me had brought.
For oft when on my couch I lie
In vacant or in pensive mood,
They flash upon that inward eye
Which is the bliss of solitude,
And then my heart with pleasure fills,
And dances with the daffodils.
    —William Wordsworth, "The Daffodils"

3. The sea is calm tonight,
 The tide is full, the moon lies fair
 Upon the straits,—on the French coast the light
 Gleams and is gone; the cliffs of England stand,
 Glimmering and vast, out in the tranquil bay.
 Come to the window, sweet is the night air!
 Only, from the long line of spray
 Where the sea meets the moon-blanched land,
 Listen! you hear the grating roar
 Of pebbles which the waves draw back, and fling,
 At their return, up the high strand,
 Begin, and cease, and then again begin,
 With tremulous cadence slow, and bring
 The eternal note of sadness in.
    —from Matthew Arnold, "Dover Beach"

4. A flock of sheep that leisurely pass by,
 One after one; the sound of rain, and bees
 Murmuring; the fall of rivers, winds and seas,
 Smooth fields, white sheets of water, and pure sky;
 I've thought of all by turns, and yet do lie
 Sleepless! and soon the small birds' melodies
 Must hear, first uttered from my orchard trees,
 And the first cuckoo's melancholy cry.
 Even thus last night, and two nights more, I lay,
 And could not win thee, Sleep! by any stealth:
 So do not let me wear tonight away:
 Without Thee what is all the morning's wealth?
 Come, blessed barrier between day and day,
 Dear mother of fresh thoughts and joyous health!
    —William Wordsworth, "To Sleep"

5. Wynken and Blynken are two little eyes,
 And Nod is a little head,

And the wooden shoe that sailed the skies
   Is a wee one's trundle-bed;
So shut your eyes while Mother sings
   Of wonderful sights that be,
And you shall see the beautiful things
   As you rock in the misty sea
Where the old shoe rocked the fishermen three:—
     Wynken,
     Blynken,
     And Nod.
     —from Eugene Field, "Wynken, Blynken, and Nod"

6. Though I speak with the tongues of men and of angels, and have not charity, I am become as sounding brass or a tinkling cymbal. And though I have the gift of prophecy, and understand all mysteries, and all knowledge; and though I have all faith, so that I could remove mountains, and have not charity, I am nothing.
   —from the Bible

7. I saw that island first when it was neither night nor morning. The moon was to the west, setting, but still broad and bright. To the east, and right amidships of the dawn, which was all pink, the day-star sparkled like a diamond. The land breeze blew in our faces, and smelt strong of wild lime and vanilla; other things besides, but these were the most plain; and the chill of it set me sneezing. I should say I had been for years on a low island near the line, living for the most part solitary among natives. Here was a fresh experience; even the tongue would be quite strange to me; and the look of these woods and mountains, and the rare smell of them, renewed my blood.
   —from Robert Louis Stevenson, *The Beach of Falesa*

8. Fourscore and seven years ago our fathers brought forth upon this continent a new nation, conceived in liberty, and dedicated to the proposition that all men are created equal. Now we are engaged in a great civil war, testing whether that nation, or any nation so conceived and so dedicated, can long endure. We are met on a great battle-field of that war. We have come to dedicate a portion of that field as a final resting-place for those who here gave their lives that that nation might live. It is altogether fitting and proper that we should do this. But in a larger sense we cannot dedicate, we cannot consecrate, we cannot hallow this ground. The brave men, living and dead, who struggled here have consecrated it far above our power to add or detract. The world will little note, nor long remember, what we say here; but it can never forget what they did here. It is for us, the living, rather to be dedicated here to the unfinished work which they who

fought here have thus far so nobly advanced. It is rather for us to be here dedicated to the great task remaining before us, that from these honored dead we take increased devotion to that cause for which they gave the last full measure of devotion—that we here highly resolve that these dead shall not have died in vain—that this nation, under God, shall have a new birth of freedom, and that government of the people, by the people, and for the people shall not perish from the earth.

   —Abraham Lincoln, Gettysburg Address

9. Then Mowgli picked out a shady place, and lay down and slept while the buffaloes grazed round him. Herding in India is one of the laziest things in the world. The cattle move and crunch, and lie down, and move on again, and they do not even low. They only grunt, and the buffaloes very seldom say anything, but get down into the muddy pools one after another, and work their way into the mud till only their noses and staring china-blue eyes show above the surface, and there they lie like logs. The sun makes the rocks dance in the heat, and the herd-children hear one kite (never any more) whistling almost out of sight overhead, and they know that if they died, or a cow died, that kite would sweep down, and the next kite miles away would see him drop and would follow, and the next, and the next, and almost before they were dead there would be a score of hungry kites come out of nowhere. Then they sleep and wake and sleep again, and weave little baskets of dried grass and put grasshoppers in them; or catch two praying-mantises and make them fight; or string a necklace of red and black jungle-nuts; or watch a lizard basking on a rock, or a snake hunting a frog near the wallows.

   —from Rudyard Kipling, *The Jungle Books*

10. Huck began to dig and scratch now. Some boards were soon uncovered and removed. They had concealed a natural chasm which led under the rock. Tom got into this and held his candle as far under the rock as he could, but said he could not see to the end of the rift. He proposed to explore. He stooped and passed under; the narrow way descended gradually. He followed its winding course, first to the right, then to the left, Huck at his heels. Tom turned a short curve, by and by, and exclaimed:

   "My goodness, Huck, looky-here!"

   It was the treasure box, sure enough, occupying a snug little cavern, along with an empty powder keg, a couple of guns in leather cases, two or three pairs of old moccasins, a leather belt, and some other rubbish well soaked with the water-drip.

   —from Mark Twain, *The Adventures of Huckleberry Finn*

10

Resonance

Human resonance is primarily brought about by the excitation of the cavities in the two airflow routes, the pharyngo-oral tract and the pharyngo-nasal passage route. The cavities may be excited by sound waves generated in the larynx or within the cavities by restricting orifices and by impounding and releasing airflow. Full fold laryngeal oscillation and valving, however, is by far the greatest source of energy for amplification in the cavities. Modulation of the airflow is made possible by the many adjustments in the sizes, shapes, couplings, openings, and wall textures of the cavities and account for the differences in energy distribution in terms of frequency and intensity of the formants that make up the various speech sounds. By modifying any of the foregoing factors that govern resonance, changes in the amplification of a sound wave can be made.

Before commencing with procedures to correct voice problems associated with cavity behaviors, the authors recommend a review of Chapter 5 and the overview material on airflow modulation in Chapter 1.

VOICE PROBLEMS ASSOCIATED WITH CAVITY SIZES AND OPENINGS

Developing Oral and Pharyngeal Resonance

EXERCISES

1. Perform the following syllable chains, attempting to increase oral and pharyngeal resonance on the vowels.
   Procedures:

(1) Relax the lower jaw and tongue.
(2) Attempt to get maximum downward movement of the mandible and tongue for the vowel.
(3) Concentrate on keeping the pharyngo-oral tract open (megaphone effect).
(4) Use good breath support; the syllables below are grouped in chains of five to encourage ample breath supply and support.
(5) Pause slightly between syllables. Pause for a normal, unhurried inhalation at the // mark.
(6) Prolong the phonemic elements of each syllable slightly.
(7) Use a downward inflection on each syllable.
a. wah-wah-wah-wah-wah // wah-wah-wah-wah-wah [wɑ]
b. waw-waw-waw-waw-waw // waw-waw-waw-waw-waw [wɔ]
c. woe-woe-woe-woe-woe // woe-woe-woe-woe-woe [woʊ]
d. yah-yah-yah-yah-yah // yah-yah-yah-yah-yah [jɑ]
e. yaw-yaw-yaw-yaw-yaw // yaw-yaw-yaw-yaw-yaw [jɔ]
f. yo-yo-yo-yo-yo // yo-yo-yo-yo-yo [joʊ]
g. rah-rah-rah-rah-rah // rah-rah-rah-rah-rah [rɑ]
h. raw-raw-raw-raw-raw // raw-raw-raw-raw-raw [rɔ]
i. row-row-row-row-row // row-row-row-row-row [roʊ]

2. The syllable chains in this exercise start from an open position. Be sure that you get your tongue and jaw in a maximum open position for the vowel before starting the syllable. Use the same procedure as is outlined in Exercise 1.
a. ahm-ahm-ahm-ahm-ahm // ahm-ahm-ahm-ahm-ahm [ɑm]
b. awm-awm-awm-awm-awm // awm-awm-awm-awm-awm [ɔm]
c. ohm-ohm-ohm-ohm-ohm // ohm-ohm-ohm-ohm-ohm [oʊm]
d. are-are-are-are-are // are-are-are-are-are [ɑr]
e. or-or-or-or-or // or-or-or-or-or [ɔr]
f. ore-ore-ore-ore-ore // ore-ore-ore-ore-ore [or]
g. ahl-ahl-ahl-ahl-ahl // ahl-ahl-ahl-ahl-ahl [ɑl]
h. all-all-all-all-all // all-all-all-all-all [ɔl]
i. old-old-old-old-old // old-old-old-old-old [oʊld]

3. This exercise is designed to bring the pharynx and mouth into greater use on syllable chains. First, practice the syllable chain with your hands cupped like a megaphone in front of your mouth. Second, practice the same chain without your hands, but pretend you are making a megaphone out of your pharyngeal and oral cavities. Open up the passageways as much as you can. Try to carry over the megaphone effect with your hands to the performance without your hands. If you can remain relaxed and maintain good quality, use a little more force without raising your pitch level.
a. ha-ha-ha-ha-ha // ha-ha-ha-ha-ha [hɑ]
b. haw-haw-haw-haw-haw // haw-haw-haw-haw-haw [hɔ]

  c. hoe-hoe-hoe-hoe-hoe // hoe-hoe-hoe-hoe-hoe [hoʊ]
  d. gah-gah-gah-gah-gah // gah-gah-gah-gah-gah [gɑ]
  e. gaw-gaw-gaw-gaw-gaw // gaw-gaw-gaw-gaw-gaw [gɔ]
  f. go-go-go-go-go // go-go-go-go-go [goʊ]
  g. rah-rah-rah-rah-rah // rah-rah-rah-rah-rah [rɑ]
  h. raw-raw-raw-raw-raw // raw-raw-raw-raw-raw [rɔ]
  i. roe-roe-roe-roe-roe // roe-roe-roe-roe-roe [roʊ]

4. Diphthongs may be used to develop greater resonance, especially since they start from an open position before moving to a more closed position on the second element. The first five chains below utilize glides in the initial position for ease in production, while the second five utilize voiced plosives in order to make the exercise more difficult. Try to get good opening of the mouth by lowering the tongue and jaw decisively on the first element of the diphthong. Try to maintain the same good quality achieved on the glides in the plosive chains.

  a. row-row-row-row-row // row-row-row-row-row [roʊ]
  b. lie-lie-lie-lie-lie // lie-lie-lie-lie-lie [laɪ]
  c. way-way-way-way-way // way-way-way-way-way [weɪ]
  d. rye-rye-rye-rye-rye // rye-rye-rye-rye-rye [raɪ]
  e. why-why-why-why-why // why-why-why-why-why [aɪ]
  f. dow-dow-dow-dow-dow // dow-dow-dow-dow-dow [daʊ]
  g. bay-bay-bay-bay-bay // bay-bay-bay-bay-bay [beɪ]
  h. down-down-down-down-down // down-down-down-down-down [daʊn]
  i. game-game-game-game-game // game-game-game-game-game [geɪm]
  j. bye-bye-bye-bye-bye // bye-bye-bye-bye-bye [baɪ]

5. Use the megaphone concept, concentrating on keeping the oral and pharyngeal passageways open, and work for maximum resonation on the following short phrases.

  a. out of them all
  b. over the cloud
  c. while calling the boy
  d. move over there
  e. high in the sky
  f. moss on the ground
  g. lawn of the mall
  h. more than I do
  i. calm as the sea
  j. role in the play

6. Try to carry over the "open mouth and throat" concept to the following sentences.

  a. "Where are you?" she cried, aiming her flashlight down the road.
  b. Our yawl rolled on the roiling waters of Balboa Bay.
  c. The moment of truth had come for Mark—either he must confront the bully now or forever be cowed by his threats.
  d. Bonnie's bouncing baby boy scowled and howled at Papa's Siamese cat.

e. The fly circled the barber's head, buzzing noisily, then landed on the end of his nose.

f. The football marathon kept the crowd glued to the TV set and dominated all New Year's Day activities.

g. "Hi, stranger!" Allen shouted, as he vaulted over the door of his sporty red car.

h. Minding one's own business might be difficult, but for friendship's sake it is an attribute to be seriously cultivated.

i. Wine became more popular in the provinces, as the price of bourbon, scotch, and rum soared.

j. Mosca, the obsequious gadfly, the servile flatterer of Volpone, is one of Ben Johnson's outstanding characters.

Sustained Resonance

The use of good liaison between words as well as the use of increased duration of vowels can do much to develop greater resonance without increasing overall force, but it has to be done properly. Duration refers to the time element involved in producing a given unit of speech (e.g., sound, syllable, word, phrase, or sentence); liaison refers to joining syllables and words within breath groups while holding intensity output at a fairly constant level. Many speakers have a tendency to decrease vocal output between syllables or words too much, allowing intensity to diminish noticeably. Compared with the speaker who uses a maximum of sustained resonance, this type of speaker generates less overall energy per phrase or sentence, even though the force used may be the same for both speakers. The person with a "choppy" delivery does not use sustained resonance, while the accomplished radio or TV announcer with his full, rich voice uses liaison to the maximum of effectiveness. Both duration of stressed syllables and smooth blending of resonance from one word to the next are of the greatest importance in producing sustained resonance.

PROCEDURES

1. Any piece of equipment that has a VU meter to monitor input can be used to study differences in intensity output of successive repetitions of speech. The procedure is described below. Exercises using the VU meter are given at the end of this section.

   (a) Set volume input dial so that the indicator needle peaks at 0 on the syllable given with maximum intensity. You can also achieve this by adjusting the distance of your mouth from the microphone —coming close to the microphone will result in an intensity increase, while moving back from the microphone will result in an intensity decrease.

   (b) During the reading, try to keep the indicator needle as close to 0 as possible; do not overdrive the system by slamming the needle beyond the 0 mark. You may have to experiment awhile before bringing your intensity level under uniform control. The clinician should model good sustained resonance for the client.

2. Developmental sentences should help to establish sustained resonance by expanding the good results obtained on a short segment to a longer one, and eventually, to the sentence as a whole. See Exercise **2** at the end of this section.

3. Experiment with the voice in reading and conversation, using a VU meter to monitor the client's intensity output. Is he able to increase intensity output on poorly delivered samples by using greater duration and sustained resonance? The selections in the last section of this chapter are suited to this type of practice.

4. Experiment with the chewing method of voice training to develop sustained resonance. The very nature of the chewing method lends itself to joining syllables in a continuous flow. The chewing method of vocal training is presented in Chapter 11. The first three phases of this program of training will assist the client to develop good resonance.

EXERCISES

1. Deliver each of the spondee words and the short sentences below twice, first with a choppy delivery; and second with a smooth, full delivery. Attempt to hold the needle on the VU meter as steady as you can throughout the utterance.

   A. Spondee words

railroad	sunshine	shipwreck	daylight
toothbrush	hardware	hayloft	firefly
bridesmaid	cupcake	mailman	downtown
barnyard	highchair	horsehide	shoeshine
cowboy	baseball	glassware	drawbridge
horseshoe	staircase	moonlight	likewise

   B. Sentences
   a. You'll find the hardware store on the corner.
   b. Old Dobbin will need a horseshoe before starting the race.
   c. The firefly will not perform in full daylight.
   d. Below freezing temperatures can cause chilblains.
   e. The moonlight on the staircase cast many long shadows in the room.
   f. At one time castor oil was a cure-all.
   g. The mailman stopped for a shoeshine when he was downtown.
   h. The shipwreck was clearly visible in the moonlight to the people on the shore.
   i. The bridesmaid will need her toothbrush after eating the cupcake.
   j. The cowboy rode across the drawbridge and into our barnyard.

k. Cheesecake, chocolate cupcakes, and strawberry shortcake were on the menu.

2. Work over each segment carefully before adding it to the rest of the sentence.

Frames	Frames
1 south wall	12 The restless mailman went downtown to buy sturdy shoes.
2 from a crack in the south wall	
3 in the hayloft came from a crack in the south wall	13 in the street
4 The sunshine in the hayloft came from a crack in the south wall.	14 ride his bicycle in the street
	15 allowed Marcie to ride his bicycle in the street
5 building supplies	16 Tommy allowed Marcie to ride his bicycle in the street.
6 has glassware and building supplies	
7 on the corner has glassware and building supplies	17 Thursday night
	18 there on Thursday night
8 The hardware on the corner has glassware and building supplies.	19 over there on Thursday night
	20 I only go over there on Thursday night.
9 sturdy shoes	21 pretty girl
10 to buy sturdy shoes	22 was a pretty girl
11 went downtown to buy sturdy shoes	23 said she was a pretty girl
	24 Everyone said she was a pretty girl.

VOICE PROBLEMS ASSOCIATED WITH CAVITY COUPLING

In Chapter 5, the various voice problems associated with inappropriate positive and negative cavity coupling are presented in detail. A review of that material is recommended before initiating the remedial procedures that follow.

PROCEDURES FOR DISCRIMINATION OF HYPERNASALITY

Frequently the person with a hypernasal voice is not fully aware of the extent of his problem, especially if it is not extreme, and needs training in discriminating between hypernasal and non-nasal sound production. Procedures 1–4 can be easily used for an operant conditioning presentation.

1. Present the following word lists (Programs I and II) to the client, hypernasalizing words randomly. The clinician should be able to model

four conditions for the client: (1) non-nasal, (2) slightly nasal, (3) nasal, and (4) very nasal. If he cannot model this range satisfactorily, he should use a recording or a skilled speaker. Have the client signal when he hears a hypernasal word. Do not go on to Procedure 2 until the client gets all of the words correct. Note that the second word list contains nasal consonants; if these are done correctly by the model, the client is not to signal. Introduce assimilation nasality on a few of the words containing nasal consonants.

Program I
Non-Nasal Words

Frames	Frames	Frames	Frames	Frames
1 badge	11 pretty	21 puppy	31 supper	41 short
2 frigid	12 bubble	22 brow	32 pry	42 rattle
3 ladies	13 bright	23 pile	33 fiddle	43 arid
4 grudge	14 stipulate	24 pole	34 putter	44 rather
5 turret	15 tulip	25 frill	35 potter	45 faceless
6 trial	16 pepper	26 fowl	36 police	46 flyer
7 felt	17 soap	27 pleasure	37 berry	47 violet
8 swell	18 power	28 brook	38 fodder	48 rough
9 further	19 goose	29 shell	39 spoke	49 crop
10 brother	20 bride	30 settle	40 surge	50 upper

Program II
Nasal and Non-Nasal Words

Frames	Frames	Frames	Frames	Frames
1 fault	11 felt	21 crumb	31 ladies	41 careless
2 sting	12 mirror	22 cruel	32 company	42 spring
3 finger	13 strutted	23 fresh	33 crop	43 English
4 growl	14 opening	24 language	34 wither	44 plumber
5 longer	15 tulip	25 fowl	35 congress	45 picture
6 torrid	16 single	26 seeping	36 jungle	46 suffer
7 tingle	17 bungle	27 remember	37 flyer	47 songster
8 rising	18 bugle	28 clue	38 bored	48 wayward
9 jungle	19 youngster	29 face	39 strength	49 supper
10 around	20 stipulate	30 frame	40 murmur	50 marrying

2. Increase the difficulty of Procedure 1 by reducing the amount of hypernasality modeled on non-nasal sounds.
3. Present the following sentences with (a) no hypernasality on non-

nasal words, (b) hypernasality on randomly selected non-nasal words, and (c) hypernasality on vowels adjacent to nasal consonants.

- a. The small craft powered its way up the river through a dense jungle.
- b. The young lad thought he would wait many years before he could consider marriage.
- c. Carelessness in the forest could mean the end of the mighty hemlocks.
- d. There wasn't a single clue to indicate who had been there.
- e. The bugler rudely blew his bugle while the company of rookies slept soundly.
- f. In the autumnal months in the mid-part of the United States the northern and southern air masses fight for supremacy.
- g. Europe is crowded with tourists in July and August.
- h. Vitamin C has been recommended for prevention of colds by some scientists, doctors, and health food advocates.
- i. From the valley floor, Sharon could see the spire of the church glistening in the sunrise.
- j. Cassie cried loud and long when Cissie whacked her knuckles.
- k. The teacher's pet in the front row always seemed to get the job of erasing the blackboard.
4. The Selections for Practice at the end of this chapter may be used to practice discrimination drills on longer passages of prose and poetry. The clinician should hypernasalize syllables, words, or phrases randomly and arrange for appropriate signals.

PROCEDURES FOR DISCRIMINATION OF PARTIAL HYPERNASALITY

Review the discussion of assimilation nasality in Chapter 5 before starting the procedures in this section.

1. Use both acoustic and tactile monitoring of the following materials. A tape recorder or Language Master should be used for review as well as critical listening during performance. The client should also place his forefinger on the side of his nose to detect the difference between nasal and non-nasal resonance. All materials are in phonetic transcription. Below is the key to the symbols used in Programs I–III that follow.
   - (a) [m-ɑ] Prolong the consonant, [m]; pause; then prolong the vowel, [ɑ]. The dash indicates a pause during which no voice is heard.
   - (b) [m:ɑ] Prolong [m], then move continuously into [ɑ]. The colon indicates a prolongation of at least one second.
   - (c) [m·ɑ] Prolong [m] half as long as in Step b, then move continuously into [ɑ]. The dot indicates about a half-second prolongation.
   - (d) [mɑ] Say [mɑ] with a good nasal and non-nasal resonance.

Note: [ŋ] does not occur in the initial position of words, but is included for drill purposes.

Program I
Initial Position of [m], [n], and [ŋ]

[m]			[n]		[ŋ]	
1 m-ɑ	9 m-u	17 n-ɑ	25 n-u	33 ŋ-ɑ	41 ŋ-u
2 m:ɑ	10 m:u	18 n:ɑ	26 n:u	34 ŋ:ɑ	42 ŋ:u
3 m·ɑ	11 m·u	19 n·ɑ	27 n·u	35 ŋ·ɑ	43 ŋ·u
4 mɑ	12 mu	20 nɑ	28 nu	36 ŋɑ	44 ŋu
5 m-ɔ	13 m-i	21 n-ɔ	29 n-i	37 ŋ-ɔ	45 ŋ-i
6 m:ɔ	14 m:i	22 n:ɔ	30 n:i	38 ŋ:ɔ	46 ŋ:i
7 m·ɔ	15 m·i	23 n·ɔ	31 n·i	39 ŋ·ɔ	47 ŋ·i
8 mɔ	16 mi	24 nɔ	32 ni	40 ŋɔ	48 ŋi

Program II
Medial Position of [m], [n], and [ŋ]

[m]			[n]		[ŋ]	
1 ɑ-m-ɑ	9 u-m-u	17 ɑ-n-ɑ	25 u-n-u	33 ɑ-ŋ-ɑ	41 u-ŋ-u
2 ɑ:m:ɑ	10 u:m:u	18 ɑ:n:ɑ	26 u:n:u	34 ɑ:ŋ:ɑ	42 u:ŋ:u
3 ɑ·m·ɑ	11 u·m·u	19 ɑ·n·ɑ	27 u·n·u	35 ɑ·ŋ·ɑ	43 u·ŋ·u
4 ɑmɑ	12 umu	20 ɑnɑ	28 unu	36 ɑŋɑ	44 uŋu
5 ɔ-m-ɔ	13 i-m-i	21 ɔ-n-ɔ	29 i-n-i	37 ɔ-ŋ-ɔ	45 i-ŋ-i
6 ɔ:m:ɔ	14 i:m:i	22 ɔ:n:ɔ	30 i:n:i	38 ɔ:ŋ:ɔ	46 i:ŋ:i
7 ɔ·m·ɔ	15 i·m·i	23 ɔ·n·ɔ	31 i·n·i	39 ɔ·ŋ·ɔ	47 i·ŋ·i
8 ɔmɔ	16 imi	24 ɔnɔ	32 ini	40 ɔŋɔ	48 iŋi

Program III
Final Position of [m], [n], and [ŋ]

[m]			[n]		[ŋ]	
1 ɑ-m	9 u-m	17 ɑ-n	25 u-n	33 ɑ-ŋ	41 uŋ
2 ɑ:m	10 u:m	18 ɑ:n	26 u:n	34 ɑ:ŋ	42 u:ŋ
3 ɑ·m	11 u·m	19 ɑ·n	27 u·n	35 ɑ·ŋ	43 u·ŋ
4 ɑm	12 um	20 ɑn	28 un	36 ɑŋ	44 uŋ
5 ɔ-m	13 i-m	21 ɔ-n	29 i-n	37 ɔ-ŋ	45 i-ŋ
6 ɔ:m	14 i:m	22 ɔ:n	30 i:n	38 ɔ:ŋ	46 i:ŋ
7 ɔ·m	15 i·m	23 ɔ·n	31 i·n	39 ɔ·ŋ	47 i·ŋ
8 ɔm	16 im	24 ɔn	32 in	40 ɔŋ	48 iŋ

2. Have the client attempt to control assimilation nasality on the following word lists, Programs I–IV. An operant conditioning approach may be used with this material.

Program I
Initial Position of [m] and [n]

[m]		[n]	
Frames	Frames	Frames	Frames
1 mat	11 map	21 nook	31 nest
2 mar	12 music	22 near	32 nose
3 meat	13 mode	23 neck	33 noose
4 most	14 mat	24 nape	34 nape
5 mill	15 much	25 neat	35 knave
6 mist	16 made	26 node	36 naive
7 meek	17 murk	27 note	37 nail
8 moot	18 moot	28 nude	38 nice
9 mark	19 more	29 next	39 night
10 mitt	20 mare	30 newt	40 nigh

Program II
Medial Position of [m], [n], and [ŋ]

[m]	[n]	[ŋ]
Frames	Frames	Frames
1 summer	21 finite	41 angle
2 simmer	22 fender	42 uncle
3 common	23 funny	43 ankle
4 dramatic	24 fence	44 canker
5 dormer	25 fancy	45 sanguine
6 tamper	26 feigned	46 anguish
7 camera	27 fringe	47 unctuous
8 temper	28 banner	48 mingle
9 seamstress	29 boner	49 tingle
10 bumper	30 phoned	50 tangle
11 clamor	31 phonic	51 finger
12 comely	32 sooner	52 fungus
13 damper	33 liner	53 linger
14 humor	34 miner	54 longer
15 dimmer	35 owner	55 singer
16 whimper	36 puny	56 bungle
17 sample	37 rented	57 shingle
18 framed	38 runic	58 trinket
19 hammer	39 toner	59 crinkle
20 loomed	40 winter	60 clunker

Program III
Final Position of [m], [n], and [ŋ]

[m] Frames	[n] Frames	[ŋ] Frames
1 dome	21 feign	41 cling
2 flame	22 own	42 sing
3 fume	23 bison	43 flung
4 room	24 piston	44 piling
5 doom	25 preen	45 soaring
6 dam	26 clean	46 belong
7 drum	27 bean	47 doing
8 blame	28 cane	48 hung
9 seem	29 chain	49 young
10 same	30 done	50 tongue
11 tomb	31 dune	51 rising
12 whim	32 fine	52 bang
13 bum	33 groin	53 king
14 comb	34 gain	54 going
15 foam	35 glen	55 morning
16 game	36 hone	56 clung
17 gleam	37 kine	57 fighting
18 gram	38 mane	58 wing
19 home	39 maiden	59 lowing
20 loom	40 foreign	60 bring

Program IV
Non-Nasal Sounds Between Nasal Consonants

One-syllable frames	Two-syllable frames	Polysyllabic frames
1 mime	1 number	1 Immanuel
2 gnome	2 mundane	2 immanent
3 moan	3 mumble	3 commemorate
4 numb	4 quinine	4 seismometer
5 mum	5 mentor	5 firmament
6 mind	6 cannon	6 demoniac
7 manx	7 remnant	7 nominal
8 mine	8 common	8 monologue
9 nine	9 mammon	9 banana
10 known	10 demon	10 ammonia
11 name	11 denim	11 immemorial
12 mane	12 nimbus	12 Camembert
13 meant	13 vermin	13 nemesis
14 man	14 nimble	14 nomenclature
15 moon	15 stamen	15 acumen
16 noon	16 gamin	16 feminine
17 nymph	17 famine	17 pneumonia
18 mint	18 venom	18 communicate
19 mink	19 lament	19 commentary
20 mend	20 bemoan	20 municipal

3. Have the client perform the following developmental sentences.

Frames	Frames
1 miner	13 knave
2 puny miner	14 young knave
3 down by the puny miner	15 fended off the young knave
4 Manley was thrown down by the puny miner.	16 The naive maiden fended off the young knave.
5 mooring	17 rhyme
6 on the mooring	18 a runic rhyme
7 to the chain on the mooring	19 by humming a runic rhyme
8 Clem clung to the chain on the mooring.	20 Sammy humored Annie by humming a runic rhyme.
9 fender	21 winter
10 Lincoln's fender	22 in summer and winter
11 clunker bumped the Lincoln's fender	23 is found in summer and winter
12 Uncle Tom's clunker bumped the Lincoln's fender.	24 The Pismo clam is found in summer and winter.

Constant Hypernasality

Review the discussion of constant hypernasility, Levels II and III in Chapter 5 before starting the procedures in this section. The discrimination exercises for hypernasality at the beginning of this section should be presented by the clinician at the outset of the training program.

PROCEDURES TO STRENGTHEN THE VELOPHARYNGEAL SEAL

If the client has marginal ability to make the velopharyngeal closure, procedures to strengthen the muscles involved in this seal may prove useful. If, however, the client is grossly unable to make this closure, this type of procedure is not indicated. Furthermore, blowing procedures *per se* do not involve precisely the same coordination of the velopharyngeal muscles as is needed for speech, or even swallowing, for that matter. Blowing continuously does little to train the timing of the closure for nasal and non-nasal speech sound combinations. For the client in need of strengthening his closure and directing his breath stream out of his mouth, the following procedures may prove useful.

1. Have the client impound the breath stream by closing the lips firmly and puffing out the cheeks. Check nasal emission by placing a steel mirror under the nostrils. Repeat several times and assign as a procedure to be repeated several times per day. Do not permit compensatory movements of the nostrils.

2. Use any type of equipment designed to measure the pressure and capacity of the client's exhalation. A wet spirometer may be used to good effect. Attempt to improve upon the best performance. Be careful not to overdo this type of activity because of the danger of introducing too much oxygen into the client's bloodstream.

3. A wide range of objects can be used in blowing exercises (e.g., feathers, pieces of tissue, Ping-Pong balls, toy soldiers, candles). Arrange the distance and objectives of the procedure to suit the client. The objects can be used in a game context for young children (e.g., playing Ping Pong soccer, blowing the object up an incline, and the like). Watch for unwanted compensatory movements carefully.

4. Place a steel mirror under the client's nose and put a feather or piece of tissue directly in front of the nostrils. Place a second piece of tissue or feather on a surface in front of the client's mouth. The client tries to blow the second feather away without disturbing the one under his nose. Distances may be increased in order to make the procedure more demanding when needed.

5. Have the client blow a series of puffs on one breath. Have him pretend he is blowing out a series of five candles, one at a time. Increase the number of candles and speed of the puffs as capacity permits. Check nasal emission and compensatory movements.

6. Have the client yawn and arch his velum as high as he can make it go. Repeat, releasing a big puff of air through the mouth. Repeat, but this time have him vocalize a breathy *ah*.

7. Have the client practice the following syllable chains, doing each one distinctly. Try to accomplish all ten syllables on one breath. Check nasal emission. Increase speed with proficiency.
   a. puh-puh-puh-puh-puh-puh-puh-puh-puh-puh [p]
   b. tuh-tuh-tuh-tuh-tuh-tuh-tuh-tuh-tuh-tuh [t]
   c. kuh-kuh-kuh-kuh-kuh-kuh-kuh-kuh-kuh-kuh [k]
   d. buh-buh-buh-buh-buh-buh-buh-buh-buh-buh [b]
   e. duh-duh-duh-duh-duh-duh-duh-duh-duh-duh [d]
   f. guh-guh-guh-guh-guh-guh-guh-guh-guh-guh [g]
   g. thuh-thuh-thuh-thuh-thuh-thuh-thuh-thuh-thuh-thuh [θ]
   h. fuh-fuh-fuh-fuh-fuh-fuh-fuh-fuh-fuh-fuh [f]
   i. suh-suh-suh-suh-suh-suh-suh-suh-suh-suh [s]
   j. shuh-shuh-shuh-shuh-shuh-shuh-shuh-shuh-shuh-shuh [ʃ]

8. Practice the following random syllable chains using the same instructions as in Procedure 7.

a. puh-tuh-kuh-buh-duh-guh-fuh-thuh-suh-shuh
b. duh-kuh-fuh-suh-tuh-shuh-buh-thuh-guh-puh
c. tuh-fuh-suh-shuh-duh-guh-kuh-puh-thuh-buh
d. duh-kuh-tuh-buh-guh-puh-fuh-shuh-thuh-suh
e. duh-fuh-suh-tuh-buh-guh-thuh-shuh-puh-kuh
f. shuh-tuh-duh-thuh-kuh-guh-suh-tuh-buh-fuh
g. kuh-fuh-thuh-buh-suh-guh-tuh-duh-shuh-tuh
h. duh-guh-kuh-suh-tuh-buh-thuh-shuh-fuh-puh
i. suh-shuh-tuh-kuh-fuh-buh-fuh-duh-puh-guh
j. tuh-duh-thuh-suh-guh-kuh-buh-shuh-fuh-puh

PROCEDURES TO ELIMINATE HYPERNASALITY ON NON-NASAL MATERIALS

Eliminating hypernasality on non-nasal materials is necessary before attempting the more difficult task of eliminating hypernasality on non-nasal speech sounds adjacent to the nasals. Several techniques described below should be used while the client is performing Exercises 1–5.

1. Use a Language Master or a tape recorder to playback the results. The client should now be taught to detect hypernasality in his own voice.
2. Monitor voiced airflow. A steel mirror placed beneath the nostrils to detect voiced airflow (by clouding) is a standard procedure and should be used. Placing feathers, tissue, and the like on a card held beneath the nose can also be helpful. Placing the forefinger adjacent to the nose (vertically over the nostrils with the fingertip on the bridge) can be used to detect voiced airflow through vibration.
3. Be aware that hypernasality does not necessarily manifest itself uniformly throughout the speech of the client. The plosives and fricatives require greater pressure and may tax the velopharyngeal seal, resulting in hypernasality. Certain vowels are more tense than others or require more pressure due to greater occlusion and therefore have a tendency to become more easily hypernasalized than others. The low back vowels ([ɑ] as in *father*, [ɔ] as in *law*, and [ʌ] as in *much*) require a low tongue position; hence, tongue and jaw positions are not as restrictive to airflow through the mouth. Use this type of vowel in developing a base line of non-nasal voice production.
4. Attempt to teach the client frontal placement. If the client has a tendency to carry his tongue and jaw high, or if he tends to occlude the oral cavity by humping up the back of his tongue, there is a possibility that the breath stream may be occluded somewhat on non-nasal sounds, resulting in hypernasality. Opening up both the pharyngeal and oral cavities and teaching frontal placement does much to eliminate hypernasality on non-nasal sounds.
5. If the client is unable to develop proper timing of the velopharyngeal

sphincter on nasal and non-nasal speech sound combinations, work on the procedures presented in the section on discrimination of partial hypernasality, see pp. 173–174.

EXERCISES WITH NON-NASAL MATERIALS

1. Occlude the nasal passages by pinching the nostrils on the first word of the following word pairs. You will note that these words do not involve high intraoral pressure. Listen carefully to the results by utilizing a Language Master or tape recorder. If a good seal has been effected, no difference in voice quality should be detected. Concentrate on frontal placement.

rear-rear	father-father	lyre-lyre
hill-hill	fir-fir	high-high
lair-lair	fall-fall	how-how
ale-ale	lure-lure	rough-rough
half-half	role-role	you-you

Repeat the word pairs, using a steel mirror placed beneath the nostrils to detect hypernasality. Were you able to complete all pairs successfully?

2. Perform the following high and low vowel word pairs. Try to retain the good results obtained on the low vowel word, which should be easiest to produce, on the more demanding high vowel in the second word of the pair. Make up other word pairs to extend this exercise.

ha-he	rah-reel	ma-me	doll-deal	shot-sheet
haw-heh	rah-lou	mall-men	tall-teal	shawl-shield
hawk-hick	wall-weal	mall-moon	pop-peat	shot-sheep
ha-heh	wall-lea	ma-mean	ball-beal	shawl-shim
haw-he	warm-weed	ma-moo	call-keel	shot-ship

Repeat the word pairs, using a steel mirror placed beneath the nostrils to detect any voiced airflow.

3. Practice the following developmental sentences, attempting to keep your voice free from hypernasality. Nasals and high pressure consonants have been kept to a minimum in order to increase the likelihood of success. Try three levels of intensity: low, medium, and medium-high (or high if it can be done successfully). Use nasal monitoring techniques to detect hypernasality. (An operant conditioning approach may be used if desired.)

Frames	Frames
1 ago	19 high at a cobalt sky
2 a week ago	20 Look up high at a cobalt sky.
3 test a week ago	21 Warren
4 Carol took her test a week ago.	22 to Warren
5 today	23 gave it to Warren
6 chariot today	24 She gave it to Warren.
7 will drive a chariot	25 Nellie
8 Tad will drive a chariot today.	26 toward Nellie
9 her	27 bounced toward Nellie.
10 about her	28 The ball bounced toward Nellie.
11 quality about her	29 mixed
12 She had a ladylike quality about her.	30 were mixed
13 record	31 cards were mixed
14 world record	32 The two decks of cards were mixed.
15 beat a world record	33 spring
16 Terry tried hard to beat a world record.	34 to the spring
17 sky	35 walked to the spring
18 cobalt sky	36 Jack and Jill walked to the spring.

4. Perform the following non-nasal sentences, using all corrective and monitoring techniques and three levels of loudness.
   a. The flower vase held a bouquet of roses with sprigs of baby's breath.
   b. Love is a powerful force for good.
   c. Prayers were offered to the Great White Spirit by the Sioux.
   d. Oaks and cedars with a few spruce covered the crest of our hill.
   e. Showers fell over the lonely desert at twilight.
   f. The pool, deep and dark, was really very clear—also cool.
   g. I could hear the wild call of the geese as they flew overhead.
   h. The blizzard tied up all the taxis.
   i. Papa blew soap bubbles to the great delight of baby Pete.
   j. Africa's areas of aridity are vast.
   k. Raspberry parfait was the featured dessert at the "Blue Fox."
   l. Our backyard was ablaze with red tulips everywhere.
   m. Fried foods irritate the gall bladder.
   n. What a fracas developed as the old feud betwixt the O'Hara brothers erupted!
   o. Blue violets hugged the shady slopes of the Frazier River.

p. The fall crops were harvested early last year.
q. Trials teach us to be grateful for periods of peace.
r. Our top discus thrower was also our top pole vaulter.
s. Oyster dishes, as well as lobster, were the specialty of the house.
t. Have you ever fished the Rogue River for steelhead?

5. Perform the following selections, attempting to eliminate hypernasality on non-nasal sounds. (Additional Selections for Practice are provided at the end of this chapter.)

a. It all started when we were driving down Pico Boulevard in metropolitan Los Angeles and spotted five brand new vacation trailers parked by a service station. Such a sight fanned the bright flame of our imaginations. Trailers, romance, the far-off places—escape from the year-round routine of congested city living. For some time we had watched and secretly envied those carefree souls who pack-up on a moment's notice and take off for points unknown, dragging their trailers behind them.

b. My heart leaps up when I behold
    A rainbow in the sky:
So was it when my life began;
So is it now I am a man;
So be it when I shall grow old,
    Or let me die!
The Child is father of the Man;
And I could wish my days to be
Bound each to each by natural piety.
        —William Wordsworth, "The Rainbow"

Hyponasality

PROCEDURES

1. Instruct the client to close his mouth and blow gently through his nasal passages. Repeat several times until the kinesthesia involved is established. Introduce voice by having the client hum a steady tone near his optimum pitch. He should then proceed as follows:

(a) Prolong an [m]. Repeat, monitoring the output by having the client place his forefinger on the bridge of his nose.

(b) Prolong an [n]. Repeat several times. Ask the client to concentrate on the kinesthetic sense, that is, tongue position, vibration, and airflow.

(c) Prolong an [ŋ]. Repeat, using the same procedure as above.

(d) Combine [m], [n], and [ŋ] with a series of vowels. Note: The colon indicates a prolongation of at least one second.

[m:ɑ]	[m:i]	[m:eɪ]	[m:æ]	[m:oʊ]
[n:ɑ]	[n:i]	[n:eɪ]	[n:æ]	[n:oʊ]
[ŋ:ɑ]	[ŋ:i]	[ŋ:eɪ]	[ŋ:æ]	[ŋ:oʊ]

Arrange for the client to move from the nasal to the vowel on a given hand signal.

2. Perform the phrases below, following these instructions: (a) Prolong the nasal consonants longer than normal; and then (b) reduce the duration of the nasal consonants to normal length.

reminded of him	fine with me
mar my face	anyone of them
many of them	loaned by him
might not go	ring no more
now and then	raining tomorrow

3. Develop the phrases in Procedure 2 into full sentences. Below are examples of typical sentences. Make up several more of your own. Have the client control the duration of the nasal consonants and keep them within the range of normal production.
   a. Jack was reminded by him.
   b. Do you think it will mar my face?
   c. Many of them will not go.
   d. Jane said that she might not go to the dance.
   e. Now and then you can hear their voices.
   f. It will be fine with me if you do it.
   g. Anyone of them can do it if they will but try.
   h. It was loaned by him to me for a month.
   i. They said that after Monday the bells would ring no more.
   j. Do you think it will continue raining tomorrow?
4. Work on the procedures contained in the section on discrimination of partial hypernasality, pp. 171–178.

DEVELOPING AWARENESS
OF THE PHONETIC POWER OF SPEECH SOUNDS

The sounds of American English vary considerably in intensity even when effort is held constant. For example, if one uses the same force to produce *aw* [ɔ] as in *law* and *th* [θ] as in *thin*, the difference in intensity between the *aw* and the *th*, as expressed by a ratio of power, is 680 to 1. An analysis of the phonetic power of speech sounds reveals that vowels and glides on the whole are relatively more powerful than plosives and fricatives, provided effort is held constant. A knowledge of the phonetic power of sounds can be valuable in developing greater vocal resonance. The table of phonetic power (Table 10.1) should be studied before beginning the exercises in this section.

Table 10.1
Intensity ratios of selected phonemes to [θ]

Phoneme	Ratio to [θ]	Phoneme	Ratio to [θ]	Phoneme	Ratio to [θ]
[ɔ]	680	[r]	210	[t]	15
[ɑ]	600	[e]	200	[g]	15
[ʌ]	510	[ʃ]	80	[k]	13
[æ]	490	[ŋ]	73	[v]	12
[ou]	470	[m]	52	[ð]	11
[ʊ]	460	[tʃ]	42	[b]	7
[eɪ]	370	[n]	36	[d]	7
[ɛ]	350	[j]	23	[p]	6
[u]	310	[dʒ]	20	[f]	5
[ɪ]	260	[z]	16	[θ]	1
[i]	220	[s]	16		

Note: The phonemes in this chart are arranged according to their phonetic power. The values are expressed in terms of a ratio, for example, [f] is five times more powerful than [θ], [ɔ] is 680 times more powerful than [θ].

EXERCISES

1. Perform the following vowels, attempting to improve resonance without increasing force. Say each vowel by itself; then, by opening your mouth a little more, manipulating your tongue position, or prolonging slightly, repeat the vowel several times until you reach maximum resonance for a given amount of force.
   a. [ɑ] as in *father*: [ɑ-ɑ-ɑ-ɑ-ɑ-ɑ-ɑ-ɑ-ɑ-ɑ]
   b. [ɔ] as in *law*: [ɔ-ɔ-ɔ-ɔ-ɔ-ɔ-ɔ-ɔ-ɔ-ɔ]
   c. [ʌ] as in *mud*: [ʌ-ʌ-ʌ-ʌ-ʌ-ʌ-ʌ-ʌ-ʌ-ʌ]
   d. [æ] as in *mat*: [æ-æ-æ-æ-æ-æ-æ-æ-æ-æ]
   e. [o] as in *obey*: [o-o-o-o-o-o-o-o-o-o]

2. Repeat the procedure in Exercise 1 with the diphthongs listed below. Observe how the resonance changes as you move from the first element of the diphthong to the second.
   a. [eɪ] as in *pay*: [eɪ-eɪ-eɪ-eɪ-eɪ-eɪ-eɪ-eɪ-eɪ-eɪ]
   b. [aɪ] as in *my*: [aɪ-aɪ-aɪ-aɪ-aɪ-aɪ-aɪ-aɪ-aɪ-aɪ]
   c. [ou] as in *low*: [ou-ou-ou-ou-ou-ou-ou-ou-ou-ou]
   d. [au] as in *now*: [au-au-au-au-au-au-au-au-au-au]
   e. [ɔɪ] as in *boy*: [ɔɪ-ɔɪ-ɔɪ-ɔɪ-ɔɪ-ɔɪ-ɔɪ-ɔɪ-ɔɪ-ɔɪ]

3. Using the same procedure as for Exercise 1, try to improve upon the resonance values of [w], [j], [l], and [r].

a. [wɑ]: [wɑ-wɑ-wɑ-wɑ-wɑ-wɑ-wɑ-wɑ-wɑ-wɑ]
b. [wɔ]: [wɔ-wɔ-wɔ-wɔ-wɔ-wɔ-wɔ-wɔ-wɔ-wɔ]
c. [wʌ]: [wʌ-wʌ-wʌ-wʌ-wʌ-wʌ-wʌ-wʌ-wʌ-wʌ]
d. [jɑ]: [jɑ-jɑ-jɑ-jɑ-jɑ-jɑ-jɑ-jɑ-jɑ-jɑ]
e. [jɔ]: [jɔ-jɔ-jɔ-jɔ-jɔ-jɔ-jɔ-jɔ-jɔ-jɔ]
f. [jʌ]: [jʌ-jʌ-jʌ-jʌ-jʌ-jʌ-jʌ-jʌ-jʌ-jʌ]
g. [lɑ]: [lɑ-lɑ-lɑ-lɑ-lɑ-lɑ-lɑ-lɑ-lɑ-lɑ]
h. [lɔ]: [lɔ-lɔ-lɔ-lɔ-lɔ-lɔ-lɔ-lɔ-lɔ-lɔ]
i. [lʌ]: [lʌ-lʌ-lʌ-lʌ-lʌ-lʌ-lʌ-lʌ-lʌ-lʌ]
j. [rɑ]: [rɑ-rɑ-rɑ-rɑ-rɑ-rɑ-rɑ-rɑ-rɑ-rɑ]
k. [rɔ]: [rɔ-rɔ-rɔ-rɔ-rɔ-rɔ-rɔ-rɔ-rɔ-rɔ]
l. [rʌ]: [rʌ-rʌ-rʌ-rʌ-rʌ-rʌ-rʌ-rʌ-rʌ-rʌ]

4. Use the same procedure for the voiced plosives [b], [d], and [g]. Experiment with the voiced implosion phase (beginning phase) of each plosive, prolonging it somewhat.
a. [bɑ]: [bɑ-bɑ-bɑ-bɑ-bɑ-bɑ-bɑ-bɑ-bɑ-bɑ]
b. [bɔ]: [bɔ-bɔ-bɔ-bɔ-bɔ-bɔ-bɔ-bɔ-bɔ-bɔ]
c. [bʌ]: [bʌ-bʌ-bʌ-bʌ-bʌ-bʌ-bʌ-bʌ-bʌ-bʌ]
d. [dɑ]: [dɑ-dɑ-dɑ-dɑ-dɑ-dɑ-dɑ-dɑ-dɑ-dɑ]
e. [dɔ]: [dɔ-dɔ-dɔ-dɔ-dɔ-dɔ-dɔ-dɔ-dɔ-dɔ]
f. [dʌ]: [dʌ-dʌ-dʌ-dʌ-dʌ-dʌ-dʌ-dʌ-dʌ-dʌ]
g. [gɑ]: [gɑ-gɑ-gɑ-gɑ-gɑ-gɑ-gɑ-gɑ-gɑ-gɑ]
h. [gɔ]: [gɔ-gɔ-gɔ-gɔ-gɔ-gɔ-gɔ-gɔ-gɔ-gɔ]
i. [gʌ]: [gʌ-gʌ-gʌ-gʌ-gʌ-gʌ-gʌ-gʌ-gʌ-gʌ]

5. Study the following sentences; underline the phonemes that have the greatest power. After you have marked the powerful sounds, perform the sentence, attempting to develop good resonance on the marked phonemes.
a. Father told Oxley to call the boys in the morning.
b. When the role was checked later in the afternoon, they found four of the soldiers gone.
c. The crowd closed in behind Roger, shouldering and pushing him to the wall.
d. Five fat rats were seen floating downstream on a log.
e. The wide end stepped out of bounds before catching the ball.
f. The commune was located in an old building in the center of the downtown area.
g. All colleges have at least one street known as Lovers' Lane.
h. Claude and Maud sought to defraud the old folks of Chapel Hall.
i. The church sexton angrily ejected the boys when he found them on the belfry tower.
j. All mankind knows the fear of lack of security; hence, the guarding of personal advantage has become second nature.

SELECTIONS FOR PRACTICE

1. Turn, Fortune, turn thy wheel, and lower the proud;
   Turn thy wild wheel through sunshine, storm, and cloud;
   Thy wheel and thee we neither love nor hate.
   Turn, Fortune, turn thy wheel with smile or frown;
   With that wild wheel we go not up or down;
   Our hoard is little, but our hearts are great.

   Smile and we smile, the lords of many lands;
   Frown and we smile, the lords of our own hands;
   For man is man and master of his fate.
   　　　　　—Alfred Lord Tennyson, "Fortune's Wheel"

2. Come, fill the Cup, and in the fire of Spring
   Your Winter-garment of Repentance fling:
   The Bird of Time has but a little way
   To flutter—and the Bird is on the Wing.

   　　　·　·　·

   O threats of Hell and Hopes of Paradise!
   One thing at least is certain—*This* Life flies;
   One thing is certain and the rest is Lies—
   The Flower that once has blown for ever dies.

   　　　·　·　·

   And that inverted Bowl they call the sky,
   Whereunder crawling cooped we live and die,
   Lift not your hands to *It* for help—for It
   As impotently moves as you or I.
   　　　　　—from Edward Fitzgerald,
   　　　　　　The Rubáiyát of Omar Khayyám

3. With fingers weary and worn,
   　　With eyelids heavy and red,
   A woman sat in unwomanly rags,
   　　Plying her needle and thread—
   　　　　Stitch! stitch! stitch!
   　　In poverty, hunger, and dirt,
   And still with a voice of dolorous pitch,
   Would that its tone could reach the rich!
   　　She sang this "Song of the Shirt!"
   　　　　　—from Thomas Hood, "Song of the Shirt"

4. Dark brown is the river,
   　　Golden is the sand,

It flows along forever,
  With trees on every hand.
Green leaves a-floating,
  Castles on the foam,
Boats of mine a-boating—
  Where will all come home?

On goes the river
  And out past the mill,
Away down the valley,
  Away down the hill.

Away down the river,
  A hundred miles or more,
Other little children
  Shall bring my boats ashore.
      —Robert Louis Stevenson,
        "Where Go the Boats?"

5. Fear death?—to feel the fog in my throat,
    The mist in my face,
When the snows begin, and the blasts denote
    I am nearing the place,
The power of the night, the press of the storm,
    The post of the foe;
Where he stands, the Arch Fear in a visible form,
    Yet the strong man must go:
For the journey is done and the summit attained,
    And the barriers fall,
Though the battle's to fight ere the guerdon be gained,
    The reward of it all.
I was ever a fighter, so—one fight more,
    The best and the last!

I would hate that death bandaged my eyes, and forebore,
    And bade me creep past.
No! let me taste the whole of it, fare like my peers,
    The heroes of old,
Bear the brunt, in a minute pay glad life's arrears
    Of pain, darkness, and cold.
For sudden the worst turns the best to the brave,
    The black minute's at end,
And the elements' rage, the fiend-voices that rave,
    Shall dwindle, shall blend,
Shall change, shall become first a peace out of pain,
    Then a light, then thy breast,

O thou soul of my soul! I shall clasp thee again,
And with God be the rest!
    —Robert Browning, "Prospice"

6. Socrates: And now, O men who have condemned me, I would fain prophesy to you; for I am about to die, and in the hour of death men are gifted with prophetic power. And I prophesy to you who are my murderers, that immediately after my departure punishment far heavier than you have inflicted on me will surely await you. Me you have killed because you wanted to escape the accuser, and not to give an account of your lives. But that will not be as you suppose: far otherwise. For I say that there will be more accusers of you than there are now; accusers whom hitherto I have restrained: and as they are younger they will be more inconsiderate with you, and you will be more offended at them. If you think that by killing men you can prevent some one from censuring your evil lives, you are mistaken; that is not a way of escape which is either possible or honourable; the easiest and the noblest way is not to be disabling others, but to be improving yourselves. This is the prophecy which I utter before my departure to the judges who have condemned me.
    —from Plato, *Apology*

7. I see millions of families trying to live on incomes so meager that the pall of family disaster hangs over them day by day.
    I see millions whose daily lives in city and on farm continue under conditions labeled indecent by a so-called polite society half a century ago.
    I see millions denied education, recreation, and the opportunity to better the lot of themselves and their children.
    I see millions lacking the means to buy the products of farm and factory and by their poverty denying work and productiveness to many other millions.
    I see one-third of a nation ill-housed, ill-clad, ill-nourished.
    But it is not in despair that I paint you that picture. I paint it for you in hope—because the nation, seeing and understanding the injustice of it, proposes to paint it out.
    —from Franklin D. Roosevelt,
    Second Inaugural Address, January 20, 1937

8. The American people are lucky in having enough men with liberal minds and keen foresight in our Government—particularly since the days of Teddy Roosevelt—to do something about the conservation of our natural resources.
    But what is conservation and what difference does it make? Who

cares? Well I care, and so does anyone else who has seen—really seen—one of our great National parks; for example, Sequoia National Park.

Sequoia, famous for its redwood trees! Trees that reach hundreds of feet into the air! Trees so wide that it takes fifteen men holding hands to completely encircle one of their trunks! So big that more than twenty five-room houses can be made from the lumber in one tree! So old that a thousand years before Christ was born they were feeling the warm rays of the sun reflecting from their green leaves and reddish branches! So magnificent that a person has to view their beauty to appreciate what nature has created!

Anyone who has climbed to the top of Morro Rock in the Sequoias cares about conservation. Morro Rock, standing several hundred feet high and perched on top of a hill, can be climbed by almost any sure-footed visitor. And what a view! Thousands and thousands of redwood trees pointing to the sky!

—from "Conservation in Our National Parks"

11

Special Procedures in Voice Training

While the easy initiation of voice production has enjoyed widespread use, other approaches, such as the chewing method, the use of sustained voice, and systematic desensitization in stimulus situations have also been employed effectively. Very little has been said about the comparative values of each method, although success has been reported for all three mentioned. Selection of method depends upon the training of the clinician, his experience and success with the procedures involved, and the responsiveness of the client to the type of training undertaken.

Certain limitations may rule out the selection of a given type of training as inappropriate. For example, if a client is unable to produce adequate phonation, attempting singing exercises would be foolish. Systematic desensitization in stimulus situations requires both extensive training for the clinician and the desire on the part of the client to engage in this type of program. But systematic desensitization in stimulus situations can be employed during and after any other approach to restoring the voice.

We do not attempt to make a comparative analysis of the strengths and weaknesses of the various approaches, but present three methods of voice training in this chapter: the chewing method of voice rehabilitation, the singing method, and systematic desensitization in stimulus situations method.

THE CHEWING METHOD

The use of the chewing method of voice training has gained widespread acceptance in vocal practice both in the United States and abroad. The method was first brought to the attention of voice clinicians by Dr. Emil Froeschels several decades ago, and, after a period of limited use, has grown in popularity among voice clinicians. The chewing method may be used either as a total program or as an adjunct to a larger program of voice training embracing more traditional methods.

The basic philosophy underlying the chewing method rests on the belief that there is a deep-rooted connection between the physiology of speaking and chewing. Froeschels has stressed the point that the central and peripheral structures involved in both these processes are essentially the same. This theory postulates that primitive man was accustomed to chewing and speaking at the same time and was not under the restraint of a strict code of manners to refrain from doing so. Furthermore, Froeschels has pointed out that babies often smack their lips after sucking and babble and gurgle while they eat.

Since eating is a biological function, it is unusual if not rare to find a person with a voice problem who is *not* relaxed while he is eating. Through the misuse of voice, or let us say, the superimposition of inappropriate behaviors upon the normal vocal processes, the person with a voice problem has departed from a more natural, inherent method of vocal production. The improper use of voice, then, eventually may lead to a breakdown in structure or function (coordination) or both.

The purpose of the chewing method is to restore the client's voice to a medium or "neutral" level characteristic of normal function. The foremost means of achieving this goal is through coupling voice production with the more primitive biological process of chewing.

PROCEDURES

Since it is difficult to determine or predict the rate of progress for a given case, the procedures are divided into four phases of activity.

PHASE I: INTRODUCTION OF CHEWING AND VOCALIZING

1. Explain the philosophy of the chewing method of voice training. If the client has adequate background instruction, resistance to the steps that follow should be at a minimum. The client will eventually develop the "correct attitude" as he achieves success through practice.
2. Demonstrate normal chewing activity with something that may be chewed easily, such as chewing gum, a crust or piece of bread, a "chewy" cookie, or the like. Ask the client to do likewise. Advise him to chew as naturally as possible and not to be self-conscious. It is important that you ask him to chew with his mouth slightly open as this discourages nasality, even though he may not do so customarily. As he is chewing ask him to be aware of the movements of the jaw, tongue, cheeks, lips, and palate. He will note that the movements are not always the same. As the morsel falls to one side or diminishes in size, the structures compensate to return it to a better position. Also, the

client will note that there is a definite front-to-back movement, which varies the process. While you don't want to make the client self-conscious or tense, you do want to make him aware of the many variations involved in chewing, and you might suggest at this point that speaking also involves many changes of a similar nature. Ask him to *feel* the entire process of chewing. This is also a good time to point out the degree of relaxation involved in the process of chewing.

3. After chewing has been established, the client should be asked to vocalize quietly while he chews, observing the following steps:

   (a) Demonstrate chewing and vocalizing for the client, using your optimum pitch level. In most cases the client will automatically use a level that is the most comfortable and natural for him. If he does not, choose an appropriate pitch level, particularly if he is too high, and ask him to lower his voice. Model the base level desired if necessary.

   (b) The voice should be inflected from the natural level, just as it is in normal speech. The client should also be encouraged to improvise pitch changes freely and should *not* be under the restraint of following a stereotyped pattern suggested by the clinician.

   (c) The vocal output of the client should be varied. As he chews the crust of bread, the chances are that he will automatically vary the movements of his articulators, and the vocal output should be a varied nonsense syllable chain. If he does not vary his chewing in any way, a repetitious syllable chain will result such as *yum-yum-yum-yum*, or *yam-yam-yam-yam-yam*. A stereotype response of this type is to be avoided; reinstruct the client, model an example or two, then ask him to try again.

   (d) Since the procedure undertaken thus far is a bit tedious, it is suggested that the clinician tape-record and play back the results for analysis in order to introduce variety. Frequent rest periods are also desirable during the early sessions.

4. Using a crust or gum, have the client chew "savagely," attempting to introduce even greater variety of vocal output into the activity. The client should concentrate more upon the movements of the articulators rather than upon increasing the intensity of the voice, as using high levels of intensity at this stage of training should be discouraged.

5. After the first session is completed, the client should be instructed to practice chewing and vocalizing two to three minutes at least once during every hour of the day. Chewing for longer practice periods can be boring and may discourage the client early in the training program.

6. The client should vary his bodily position during practice both in the clinic and at home. He should be able to demonstrate success on all steps, while seated, lying down, or walking. He should be encouraged to relax in all postures.

7. There are several criteria for judging success of the chewing method of voice rehabilitation that should be utilized in instruction:
   (a) The client uses a pitch level that is appropriate for his voice.
   (b) The vocal output of the client reveals few syllable repetitions.
   (c) The client's voice quality shows some improvement in nonsense vocalization over his speaking quality at this stage of therapy.
   (d) The client chews and vocalizes with relative abandonment. It is important that the movements be done freely and easily, which is characteristic of the biological function of eating.
   Note: The chewing method has one distinct advantage over traditional methods of training the voice at the initial stage of work, namely, that the client can practice with little threat of damage to the vocal structures. He should be encouraged to practice several times a day after the first session.

PHASE II: INTRODUCTION OF IMAGINARY CHEWING OF PHRASES

1. After the preliminary phase of using a piece of gum or crust of bread and establishing good variety of vocalized nonsense syllables, have the client *imagine* he is chewing while he vocalizes. If he is unable to make the transition smoothly, reintroduce the crust of bread to establish a base line of performance, then follow this step with imaginary chewing and vocalization. Using a tape recorder for replay and analysis will help the client to detect differences between the two steps.
2. Ask the client to chew "savagely" after the procedure established in Phase I, Step 4, but this time with an imaginary morsel.
   Note: Instruction at this point may follow two modes, modeling and shaping. If the client lapses into a repetitious or monotonous pattern, interrupt him and demonstrate the correct pattern. You may also pre-arrange a signal designating that he is beginning to do the procedure correctly, then remove the signal (finger, light, or the like) when he lapses into the incorrect pattern. He is instructed to try to achieve greater periods of success.
3. Introduce meaningful speech. Explain to the client that speech is a constant flow of syllable chains rather than a "chopped up" series of words. The diagnosis will have revealed the degree to which the patient utilizes liaison of words in his every day speech. Demonstrate easy syllable flow for the client. The section on the use of sustained resonance in Chapter 10 may be helpful in explaining this concept.
   (a) Have the patient chew and vocalize a few short nonsense phrases of his own, for example, [jʌmʃoʊleɪmi], [gaboʊjaði]. Instruct him to make them easily and effortlessly without giving him a precise model or instructions. It is important that he improvise on his own. The clinician may model or explain what he wants in terms of ease and length of the sample, however.

(b) Have the client chew and say the following phrases and short sentences:

in the house	I'm over here.
out of here	Where are you?
have you seen	How high is it?
the one on the corner	I'm glad to meet you.
the boy with the ball	He went to the store.

It is better to work on each phrase or sentence, attempting to retain good vocalization while fading the chewing somewhat, rather than reading the phrases and sentences in a series without interruption. If the transition between nonsense vocalization and phrase production is erratic, move back one step in order to reestablish proper rendition of the nonsense material rather than asking for many repetitions of a poorly done phrase. Likewise, if voice quality remains poor, it is better to stay on nonsense material and vary production attempts between chewing a real morsel and an imaginary one.

4. Many clients will have a tendency to become hypernasal while chewing and vocalizing. In order to prevent hypernasality, try the following procedures:

(a) *Yawning.* Have the client yawn and move into nonsense vocalization while chewing. The yawn is effective in initiating a non-nasal utterance.

(b) *Shaping.* Signal the client when he is non-nasal; attempt to increase the amount of non-nasal production.

(c) *Discrimination.* The clinician models inappropriate hypernasality intermittently with non-nasal production. The client signals when inappropriate hypernasality is heard. Have the client make a tape recording, then analyze the recording for inappropriate hypernasality.

5. Apply the same criteria for success on Phase II as was used for Phase I (see Step 7).

PHASE III: TRANSITION TO MEANINGFUL MATERIAL

Some clients have difficulty in making a smooth transition from nonsense chewing to meaningful speech. Attain mastery on one step before moving on to a more advanced level.

1. Establish a base line of good nonsense vocalization and chewing. After this has been done, perform Phase II, Step 3. Fade the amount of chewing somewhat, attempting to retain the same quality of performance.

2. Work on the following rhythmical lines and short selections, observing these guidelines:

(a) At first, do only one line at a time.

(b) Alternate the line with a nonsense syllable chain about the same length.

(c) Use a similar rhythm, pitch, and syllable pattern on the nonsense material as is contained in the line.

(d) Fade the chewing movements on both the nonsense chain and the meaningful line.

(e) Attempt to maintain good vocal output on longer segments of material.

(f) Move back to nonsense material and more active chewing if vocal production is unsatisfactory.

(g) The use of a tape recorder for analysis is highly recommended.

(h) Use frequent rest periods.

a.   Sing a song of sixpense
     A pocket full of rye
     Four and twenty blackbirds
     baked in a pie.
          —from *Mother Goose*

b.   I told them once, I told them twice.
     They would not listen to advice.

c.   "The time is come," the Walrus said,
     "To talk of many things:
     Of shoes—and ships—and sealing wax—
     Of cabbages—and kings—
     And why the sea is boiling hot—
     And whether pigs have wings."
          —from Lewis Carroll, *Through the
          Looking-Glass*

d.   The sea! The sea! the open sea!
     The blue, the fresh, the ever free!
          —Bryan Waller Proctor, "The Sea"

e.   The little cares that fretted me,
     I lost them yesterday
     Among the fields above the seas,
     Among the winds at play. . . .
          —from Elizabeth Barrett Browning,
          "Out in the Fields"

f.   Water, water, everywhere
     And all the boards did shrink;
     Water, water, everywhere,
     Nor any drop to drink. . . .
          —from Samuel Taylor Coleridge,
          "The Rime of the Ancient Mariner"

g. Breathes there the man with soul so
        dead
    Who never to himself hath said;
    This is my own, my native land!
        —from Robert Burns

h. The Moving Finger writes; and,
        having writ,
    Moves on: nor all your Piety nor
        Wit
    Shall lure it back to cancel half
        a Line,
    Nor all your Tears wash out a
        Word of it.
        —from Edward Fitzgerald,
        The Rubáiyát of Omar Khayyám

i. Tell me not in mournful numbers
    Life is but an empty dream.
    For the soul is dead that slumbers,
    And things are not what they seem.
        —from Henry Wadsworth Longfellow,
        "A Psalm of Life"

j. At one moment the light is not seen; it is overcast with clouds
    and rain; then the wind passes by and clears them away, and
    a golden glow comes from the north.

3. Using the same procedure as in Step 2, work on the following lines.
    a. In the twilight hours of evening the fireflies come a-wooing.
    b. Oh, where are you going my little friend?
    c. The South Wind said that the North Wind was the stronger of the
        two.
    d. In the days to come the lion and the lamb shall lie down together,
        and peace shall reign on earth.
    e. The light of the cave was dim, but the boys could make out a path-
        way through the dark.
    f. He waved to the girls on the shore, but they were too preoccupied
        with the handsome lifeguard to notice.
    g. Harold and Harvey were running across the field when the balloons
        were released in the stadium.
    h. Never throw trash on the highways nor pollute our streams.
    i. Let us all work together to keep the balance of nature.
    j. Let us regard our environment with reverence.
    k. He faked to the running back, rolled out toward the north sidelines,
        then threw a long pass into the end zone.
    l. Blewett lined up his putt with all the precision of an engineer,

calmly took his position over the ball, then with the touch of a master stroked the pellet five feet past the hole.

4. Use the criteria for success described in Phase I, Step 7.
5. Ask the client to practice nonsense chewing for two to three minutes every hour. He should now set aside at least ten to fifteen minutes for practice of meaningful material, provided he can demonstrate control and can self-monitor production. He should know how to move backward to achieve base line quality if vocal production is inadequate.

PHASE IV: TRANSITION TO EVERYDAY SPEECH

1. Establish a base line of good nonsense chewing. Perform the exercises described in Phases II and III, maintaining good control of vocal production.
2. Have the client read several of the Selections for Practice at the end of Chapters 8 and 9. Use whatever procedures are needed to maintain satisfactory vocal output.
3. Engage the client in conversation. Use topics that evoke responses readily. The following material may be expanded by the clinician and the client as suits the occasion.
   A. Short questions and answers:

a. How are you?	I'm fine, thank you. How are you?
b. Where are you going?	I'm going to the store to get some cards.
c. What are you looking for?	I'm looking for the keycase you gave me last Christmas.
d. What are you doing now?	I'm working for a broker in the University district.
e. What is the easiest way to go?	If I were going and were given my choice, I would drive rather than take a bus.
f. Where is the closest gas station from here?	I don't know; I'm a stranger here myself!
g. What kind of car are you driving now?	I sold my car last fall, and I don't plan to get another one for some time.
h. How old are you?	You really shouldn't ask, but since you did, let's say I'll be thirty-nine on my next birthday!
i. What time is it?	Check with the clock on my desk—it's more accurate than my wristwatch.
j. Can you go to lunch?	I'd like to very much, but I'll have to be back early.

   B. Ask questions requiring longer responses:
   a. Tell me something about the nature of your work.

b. What is your favorite hobby?
c. What do you like about travel? Restaurants?
d. What are your impressions about foreign travel? Modern Painting? Architecture?
e. What kind of food do you like best?
f. What is your favorite kind of music? Why?
g. What is your favorite sport? Why?
h. Who do you think will be the next President of the United States?
i. Do you feel graduate education needs revision?
j. Discuss some of your favorite books and authors.
C. Engage the client in short, impromptu discussions on subjects of contemporary interest.

Try to keep the discussion as spontaneous as possible. Work for frequent exchanges of communication. Give instructions for modification of the client's output after conversational units have been completed, or at appropriately timed opportunities, rather than interrupting the natural flow of conversation. Signaling, fading, chewing, and shaping, as well as other correctional techniques, may be used at this time.

SUSTAINED PHONATION OR SINGING APPROACH

If the client is able to sustain voice production and has the ability to sing, both clinician and client might consider the sustained voice approach to training as a means of developing greater vocal endurance, flexibility, and better quality.

Many voice clinicians use humming to place the voice, but do little more with singing than using just this one technique. Many of our clients rely heavily upon their voices for vocational purposes (lawyers, teachers, salesmen, entertainers) and really need a program of strengthening the voice after restoration in order to meet the unusual demands of their professions. A program of singing exercises, for those who can do them, is ideally suited as an adjunct to vocal rehabilitation, in that, in terms of endurance, it can give the client a little more margin to work with than he had before. It would seem, then, that if we would seek to give our clients greater ease and efficiency in producing voice at the vocal fold level, some consideration might be given to singing exercises.

Symptoms of Vocal Deterioration in Singing

The following symptoms are characteristic of singers suffering voice breakdowns: (a) inability to sustain and diminish high notes; (b) inability to control pitch breaks; (c) inability to diminish or sustain voice at lower levels of intensity; (d) loss of a *ringing* or *bell-like* quality; and (e) fatigue or breakdown of voice during performance.

Goals

The singing approach to vocal rehabilitation stresses the following goals: (a) producing tone with ease throughout the singing range; (b) training in the production of tone at low levels of intensity (piano and pianissimo); (c) development of flexibility of the voice; (d) working on pitch breaks by initiating tone above the break (in pitch) and moving continuously through and below the breaking point; (e) training in diminishing tones that are fully supported to falsetto without breaks or *clicks*; (f) development of a *ringing* type of resonance; (g) development of a steady tone (as opposed to voice with a pronounced vibrato or tremulo); (h) development of powerful, "easy to produce" high notes; and (i) spreading of good resonance from one part of the range to another.

Guidelines for Using the Singing Approach

Not all clients are suited for the singing approach to voice training. It is important that the clinician explain the approach in detail before deciding to employ it. The following guidelines may be applied to determine the advisability of using singing exercises with clients.

1. After appropriate explanation of the method, the client should elect and be willing to pursue a program of singing exercises. Motivation is one of the most vital keys to success in the singing approach. If the client does not like to sing, has little aptitude for it, or does not want to sing, it is folly to urge that he undergo a rather intensive program of singing exercises.

2. The client should be able to sustain voice on a given pitch. He may not be able to do so at the outset of training; therefore, singing exercises may have to be postponed until later in the remedial program.

3. The client should be able to perform exercises on key as well as singing them accurately after rehearsal. Many clients cannot accomplish even the simplest exercise and therefore are poor candidates for this type of training.

Singing exercises should be considered as an adjunct to regular voice training rather than a total method in itself. Singing exercises, for those who can perform them, are very useful in developing vocal strength. Clients who have vocational demands upon their voices, such as teachers, ministers, salesmen, actors and others, may find singing exercises, properly executed, an excellent way to build up their vocal endurance.

Before beginning the exercises in this section, study Table 11.1 to familiarize yourself with musical symbols, terms, and descriptions.

PROCEDURES

The clinician should use a pitch pipe, piano, or a taped model of the musical exercise for all of the procedures in the three phases of training.

Table 11.1
Glossary of Terms

Term	Symbol	Description
piano	p	soft
pianissimo	pp	very soft
mezzo forte	mf	medium loud
forte	f	loud
crescendo	$<$	gradually increasing loudness
diminuendo	$>$	gradually decreasing loudness
legato	leg	smooth; no interruption between notes

The clinician should also be able to model all musical exercises, as well as being able to correct the client when he does not perform satisfactorily.

PHASE I: LIMBERING AND FLEXIBILITY EXERCISES

1. Flexibility exercise:

Flexibility Scale

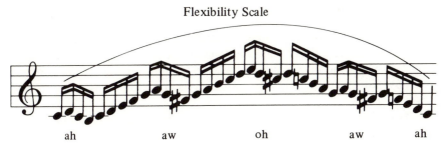

ah   aw   oh   aw   ah

Keys: A♭, A, B♭, B, C, D♭

  (a) Hum lightly the above scale. Practice the turns if they are difficult to manage at first (e.g., F-G-A-G-F♯-G-A, C-D-E-D-C♯-D-C, and A-G-A-G-F♯-G-F). Be sure to hum pianissimo throughout. If you cannot sustain tone at a low level of loudness, select the lowest level of intensity that you can do successfully, then work for a softer tone.
  (b) Sing the entire exercise on the vowel [i] in one breath. Keep the tone pianissimo throughout the exercise. Attempt to relax your entire vocal mechanism. You should eventually do this exercise at a rate of four or five notes per second.
  (c) Repeat the exercise using the vowels *ah, aw,* and *oh,* as indicated. Blend smoothly from one vowel to the next and keep the intensity pianissimo at all times.

(d) Repeat steps (a-c) on the keys indicated below the scale. It is probably best to start with the lowest key, A♭, and work up to the highest, D♭. Don't strain at any time.

Note: This exercise is excellent for limbering up and should be used in three ways: (1) limbering up before doing other exercises; (2) relaxing and limbering up after doing sustained or more forceful vocal exercises; and (3) removing phlegm from vocal cords.

2. Tone-building exercise:

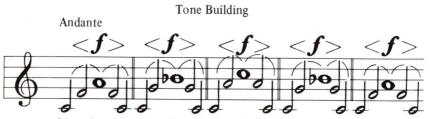

Tone Building

ah aw oh aw ah ah aw oh aw ah ah aw oh aw ah ah aw oh aw ah ah aw oh aw ah

Keys: C, B, B♭, D♭, D

(a) Hum lightly, increasing the loudness slightly as the high note is reached, then swelling the tone in a pronounced crescendo, after which the tone is diminished and slurred down to the base level.

(b) Sing [i] using the same instructions regarding crescendo-diminuendo.

(c) Sing the vowels *ah, aw,* and *oh* as marked. Attempt to gain a "ringing" tone quality on the high note.

(d) Work on A, B♭, and B. No more than five minutes total time should be spent on this demanding exercise. You may elect to start on the lowest key and work toward the highest.

3. Resonance-developing exercise:

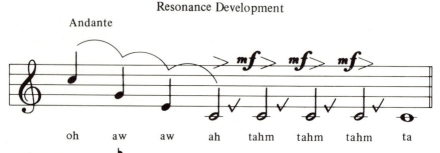

Resonance Development

oh   aw   aw   ah   tahm   tahm   tahm   ta

Keys: C, B, and D♭
Note: ✓ indicates a catch breath.

(a) Sing the octave from C to C on the intervals indicated, using the vowels *oh, aw,* and *ah.* Work for evenness of resonance and slur from note to note.

(b) On separate breaths, sing three *tahm*'s, as indicated, then sustain a final *ta.* Start each syllable with a moderate amount of force (mf) and diminish them to pianissimo.

(c) Repeat several times. It is wise to limit the amount of time spent working on lower pitch levels with force. Such a practice has a tendency to decrease the ease of producing resonance in the upper range in the attempts that may immediately follow. Also, many persons whose voices have been fully developed in the middle range first have had difficulty in developing upper range resonance later.

PHASE II: BUILDING RESONANCE

After Phase I has been satisfactorily established, go on to Phase II exercises (pp. 204–206), using the following procedure.

1. Use Phase I musical exercises to limber up the voice, especially the flexibility exercise. Then introduce the interval scale exercise, below. Rehearse it until the client is able to do it without prompting. Repeat, then rest a few minutes before continuing with the nonsinging part of the clinical session. Assign the interval scale exercise to the daily practice sessions to be done away from the clinic. These practice periods at home (or elsewhere) should be short, not lasting more than ten to twelve minutes. It is better to practice twice for a ten-minute period than once for twenty minutes; it is better to practice three times a day for ten minutes each than to drill for fifteen minutes twice, and so on.

2. Use Phase I exercises to limber up the voice, especially the flexibility scale. Then perform the first Phase II exercise, the interval scale. Introduce the second Phase II exercise. Rest before continuing with the nonsinging vocal work. Assign the second Phase II exercise to the home drill program.

3. After preliminary exercises to limber up the voice, add the third Phase II exercise to the program. Assign this exercise to be done in the home drill program. Continue with your nonsinging voice work in the clinic. The clinician may elect to eliminate the second and third Phase I exercises, in order to shorten the drill period in the clinic. At this time the clinician is more interested in maintaining and improving the client's voice quality than he is in doing all of the exercises in every phase. He is also aware that the client will have more time for practice at home than he will in the clinic; therefore, as the number of exercises in the repertoire grows, greater selectivity of which ones to perform becomes important. The clinician must outline the exercises he wants the client to perform within the ten-minute drill periods at home, particularly

during the first two phases of training. The home training program becomes more important as the client progresses, as the building of strength in a voice depends on regular daily drills performed correctly. The instruction in the clinic can only guide the client in how to perform the exercises correctly; the degree of progress is in direct ratio to the amount of work done away from the clinic.

EXERCISES

1. Interval-scale exercise:

Interval–Scale Octave

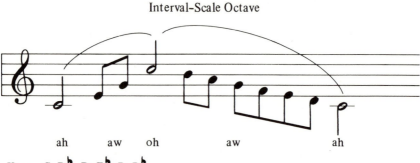

ah   aw   oh   aw   ah

Keys: C, D♭, D, E♭, B, B♭

(a) Hum the intervals, C-E-G-C, then return on the continuous scale B-A-G-F-E-D-C. Keep the tone piano-pianissimo. Move continuously and easily through the scale on one breath.

(b) Repeat step (a) using the vowel [i]. Be sure to keep the tone pianissimo and complete the scale in one breath.

(c) Use the vowels *ah, aw,* and *oh* as indicated. Keep the tone "light" and get good liaison from one note to the next. Repeat, if necessary, to improve on your performance.

(d) Repeat steps (a-c) on the keys indicated below the scale.

2. Octave-interval exercise:

Octave–Interval

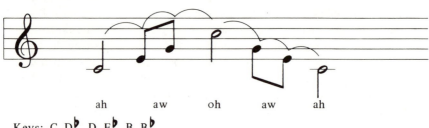

ah   aw   oh   aw   ah

Keys: C, D♭, D, E♭, B, B♭

(a) Perform the octave C-C, using the intervals E and G.
(b) Hum the scale first at the pianissimo level. Hold the half-notes longer than the quarter notes. Attempt to move continuously and easily from one note to the next in a "slurring" way. Repeat if necessary.
(c) Repeat step (b) on the vowel [i]. Be sure to keep the tone pianissimo. Slightly more loudness may be used on the upper C if the tone has a tendency to break.
(d) Sing the scale with the vowels *ah, aw,* and *oh* as marked. Try to maintain ease of production and clarity of tone.
(e) Repeat steps (a-d) in the keys of Db, D, Eb, B, and Bb if the results on C have been satisfactory.

3. Developing upper-range resonance:

Upper–Range Resonance

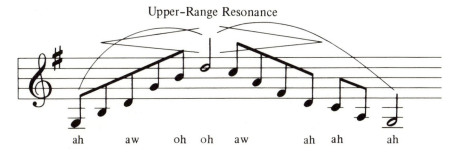

ah   aw   oh   oh   aw   ah   ah   ah

Keys: G, A♭, A

(a) Hum the scale as written. Sing piano and increase the loudness gradually to mf as you approach the high note; return to the low note as indicated, decreasing loudness gradually to piano.
(b) Repeat step (a) on the vowel [i].
(c) Sing the scale using *ah,   aw,* and *oh* with increasing loudness from mf at the beginning to F on the high note, then decrease loudness (diminuendo) on the return to the low note.

4. Developing upper-range resonance and flexibility:
(a) Sing the vowels as indicated.
(b) Sing the first note in a short burst; diminish it crisply. Sing the second note (an octave higher) crisply (a very short crisp *ho*); however, let a little breath escape on the *h.* The entire exercise is to be sung forte.
(c) Sing down the scale briskly as indicated.
(d) After reaching the bottom note, quickly move to the next note higher without terminating the tone.

Upper Resonance and Flexibility

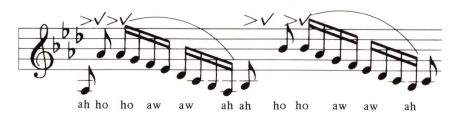

ah ho   ho   aw   aw   ah ah   ho   ho   aw   aw   ah

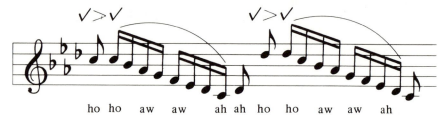

ho ho   aw   aw   ah ah ho   ho   aw   aw   ah

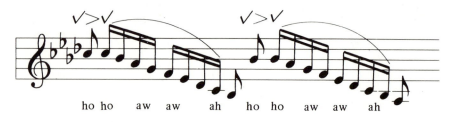

ho ho   aw   aw   ah   ho ho   aw   aw   ah

Keys: A♭, A, B♭, B
Note: √ indicates a catch breath.

- (e) Complete the rest of the exercise. Notice the progressively cyclical nature of this exercise, which leads you back to the note you began on.
- (f) Perform all steps (a-e) in the key of A. Do likewise for the key of B♭ and B.

PHASE III: STRENGTHENING THE VOICE

This group of exercises is designed to build a full and powerful voice in the upper range; the exercises should be approached with caution. Since the upper range is much less involved in speaking than in singing, it is not necessary to embark on this phase of training for speaking purposes. If the clinician and client elect to continue with the singing program, Phase III should be begun only after Phase II has been mastered. You will note that the exercises demand sustained high notes, which may be difficult for the client to accomplish at first. The client must not force his vocal output at any time. Add one exercise at a time, and observe the instructions carefully. Since the repertoire of exercises is now too large to include all of them in the practice sessions, the clinician must make a judicious selection of exercises for drill both in the clinic and at home. It is always wise after finishing a forte or double forte exercise to practice the first exercise of Phase I and then rest (or, better, rest, and then do the exercise).

EXERCISES

1. Interval approach to sustained high note:

Sustained High Note from Interval Approach

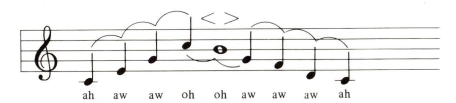

ah   aw   aw   oh   oh   aw   aw   aw   ah

Keys: C, D♭, D, B, B♭, A

(a) Hum up the scale lightly, sustaining the whole note as indicated before returning down the scale. Use a legato, joining vowels with a slight additional emphasis on successive notes. Increase the loudness on the climax note (crescendo), then diminish it before returning back down the scale.

(b) Repeat step (a) on the vowel [i].

(c) Sing the vowels *ah, aw,* and *oh* as indicated. Increase and decrease the loudness of the *oh* in a crescendo-diminuendo before returning to beginning note. The exercise should commence with *ah* being sung piano, and the loudness should be increased gradually until the highest note is reached. Then the tone should be *slurred* into the climax note and increased to the forte level by the time the whole note is half way finished. Work for a ringing quality. *Do not force the voice.*

(d) Repeat the entire procedure on the other keys. Work up to a time maximum of five minutes. Each step can be repeated until the clinician feels the client has achieved the results he needs to go on. The exercise should be terminated if unsatisfactory results persist.

2. Tone building in the upper range:

(a) Hum the octave intervals C-C very lightly (pianissimo). Repeat if needed.

(b) Sing the octave interval, C-C, using *ah* on the low note and *me,*

Tone Building in Upper Range

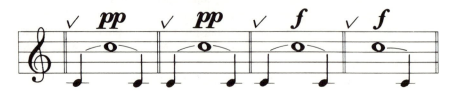

Keys: C, D♭, D, B, B♭
Note: ∨ indicates a catch breath.

me, me, me on the high note, then returning to *ah* on the low note. Sing pianissimo at all times, attempting to get a good focus (tone adjustment) on the *me*'s, which are repeated several times. Repeat if necessary to improve your performance.

(c) Sing *ah* on the low note and *me-you-oh* on the high note, sustain the *oh* a moment, then return to the *ah* on the low note. Sing forte throughout, but don't force the tone. Blend the *me-you-oh* smoothly and continuously, attempting to open up into a fully resonated *oh* before returning to base level. The *me-you* portion of the phrase attempts to focus the tone before opening up for the *oh*.

(d) Sing *oh* (on the high note for one and a half to two seconds and return to the low note *ah* [ɑ]. Repeat several times attempting to get a well-resonated *oh* on the high note.

3. Developing middle- and upper-range resonance:

Middle- and Upper-Range Resonance

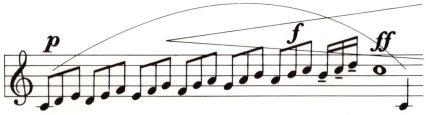

ah ah oh ah ah oh ah ah oh awaw oh aw aw oh aw oh oh oh oh oh   oh   ah

Keys: C, D♭, D, E♭, B, B♭

(a) Hum the entire exercise lightly (pianissimo).
(b) Sing the exercise using the vowel [i].
(c) Sing the exercise as indicated (*ah, aw, oh,* and so on) in the fol-

lowing manner: First, sing the first three triplets (9 notes) lightly, phrasing the triplets by slight emphasis. Then sing the next twelve notes in a similar manner but increase loudness until you reach the sustained climax note; observe the vowels to be sung. Stress the last triplet of *oh*'s as indicated. Then finish by diminishing the climax note and return to low C.

(d) Repeat steps (a-c) on the other keys indicated.

THE USE OF SYSTEMATIC
DESENSITIZATION IN STIMULUS SITUATIONS

A number of voice clinicians have applied the principle of reciprocal inhibition to stimulus situations in carefully constructed hierarchies involving encounters that produce negative emotion to modify the vocal behavior of patients with voice disorders. The approach should be familiar to those who know the work of Wolpe, Lazarus, and others; this method of behavior modification has been used extensively by speech pathologists, particularly in the area of stuttering.

The chief focus of training is upon the circumstances surrounding the improper use of voice, especially those situations where negative emotion is present, rather than upon the voice itself. Before launching into training, the clinician would be wise to explain the procedure in some detail to the client to ascertain whether or not he wishes to participate in this type of vocal rehabilitation. Systematic desensitization procedures can be used as a total approach to voice training, or they can be used after adequate voice production has been established by direct approaches.

While the underlying principles and procedures of the use of systematic desensitization in stimulus situations are clear-cut and not difficult to understand, their application requires considerable skill on the part of the clinician and persistence and dedication on the part of the client.

Analysis of Stimulus Situations

The initial stage of therapy should be focused upon identifying and gathering information concerning the situations that produce negative emotion for the client. While the diagnostic interview presented in Chapter 2 will be helpful in providing a format for obtaining important information about the voice problem, a systematic study of the situations producing negative emotion is best conducted with a speech situation checklist. The Iowa Stutterer's Self-Ratings of Reactions to Speech Situations, Form 16, is typical of this type of checklist. Brutten and Shoemaker have developed a more extensive questionnaire of speech situations that often involve negative emotion.[1] It is also possible to develop a checklist for the client based on case history materials.

The checklist should be used as the format for extensive interviewing. The information obtained from the interviews will be very helpful in aiding the client to order increments of the amount of negative emotion within a hierarchy from least to greatest. The analysis of the stimulus situations producing negative emotion will take several sessions involving considerable self-analysis by the client before hierarchy construction can begin.

Teaching Reciprocal Inhibition

This step may begin immediately along with interviewing. Usually, six or more sessions with considerable homework are required before the clinician can attempt to apply reciprocal inhibition to the steps on the hierarchies. According to Wolpe, negative emotion will be greatly reduced or absent in the presence of a well-established reciprocal inhibitor, such as deep relaxation, assertive behavior, positive emotional responses, or the like.[2] One should ask the question, "What produces a positive response in the client?" For a child, it may be the thought of eating ice cream. For an adult, it may be scenes of pastoral beauty, sailing a boat, or hitting a beautiful golf shot. Ask the client to give you a list of things he enjoys or reacts to most favorably. These should be used to inhibit negative emotion. Progressive relaxation, hypnosis, forms of suggestion, and assertive behavior may also be used as the reciprocal inhibitor. Do not begin systematic desensitization training until the reciprocal inhibitor is well established and can be readily demonstrated by the client. See Chapter 7 for procedures in teaching relaxation.

Hierarchy Construction

The information obtained from the personal interviews should now be arranged into hierarchy categories. Wolpe has recommended that at least four different themes be developed, e.g., talking to persons in authority; talking to people in sales meetings, or group gatherings; talking to people who are unsympathetic or dominant; and so forth.

The arrangement of the steps or scenes in the hierarchy is often a time-consuming task, since the steps must be ordered in terms of difficulty. According to Wolpe, the increments between steps should be fairly uniform, that is, the difference in negative emotion amount between steps 1 and 2 should be approximately the same as between steps 5 and 6. The total num-

[1] Eugene J. Brutten and L. M. Webster, "The Modification of Stuttering and Associated Behaviors," in *Communication Disorders: Remedial Principles and Practices,* ed. Stanley Dickson (New York: Scott, Foresman, 1974).
[2] J. Wolpe, *Psychotherapy by Reciprocal Inhibition* (Stanford: Stanford University Press, 1958).

ber of steps to be developed for any one theme may vary, depending on the strength of the negative emotion developed by the situation. An average of 12 to 15 steps is suggested. More steps may be added if the gradient between steps is found to be too steep. The salient details of each step must be carefully considered, as the client must supply these features to the clinician for presentation.

The clinician must be careful not to lead the client in determining the order of scenes. Clients often report that the strength of the negative response varies according to a number of variables (such as the circumstances of a particular day or a response to a particular individual). This suggests that the clinician must be constantly on the alert to detect problems that might develop with regard to the sequential arrangement of the hierarchy.

Presenting the Scenes

The room, the absence of competing stimuli, and the manner in which the scenes are presented are of importance in carrying out the training program. The room should be reasonably quiet, the client should be comfortably seated, and it is probably best for the clinician to be out of the line of vision of the patient. In many clinics, clinicians prefer to present the scenes through a speaker system from a second room with a one-way viewing screen. Words and sentences used by the clinician to present the scenes must be carefully considered, as they constitute the stimuli that trigger the scene in the mind of the client. One need not give all of the details of a scene, as the client supplies most of the details by interjecting himself into the situation. Sensory details are important in presenting verbal clues. The time for each presentation should be of short duration, but can vary from a few seconds up to fifteen seconds or more, depending on the nature of the scene. The time between scenes should be held relatively uniform, from fifteen to twenty seconds. Remember, the client is instructed to signal the clinician if a negative response has occurred. A signal button and light or a hand signal for the client will serve satisfactorily as the means of communication.

The sequence of presentation of scenes is from the least negative emotional response produced to the greatest. The first scene is presented; if no anxiety signal is given by the client, the scene is repeated, using uniform intervals for scene presentation and silent recall (e.g., seven to ten seconds for presentation and twenty seconds for recall). After the second successful recall period without a negative response signal, the clinician should go to the next scene.

If the client flashes a negative response, dissolve the scene by assuring him that he is in the clinic room, safe, and that he should attempt to relax once more and be comfortable. It is important to back up at least one scene and reinstate two successful presentations before attempting the scene that produced the negative emotional response again. If the gradient is too

steep between scenes, the clinician may have to develop new, easier steps, or move the difficult scene further along in the hierarchy.

Scenes may be presented visually as well as auditorily, or in both ways. A series of slides depicting typical speech situations can be arranged in order of difficulty. For example, a slide showing a woman seated at a desk could serve as a stimulus. You may tell the client that he is approaching this person and eventually will initiate conversation. You might say that the woman is a receptionist for a business firm. The point is that the client interjects himself into the situation without the clinician having to say much about it. Situations involving a wide range of life experiences can serve as sources for scenes (e.g., ordering at a restaurant, grocery store encounters, social gatherings, and the like). Clients usually project themselves into the situations with a high degree of realism and reaction. Videotapes can also be made and used to good advantage to present the series of graded scenes.

Behavior Rehearsal

As in all therapy, the most difficult step is to move from the carefully controlled laboratory experiments to the variable world of reality. As a means of bridging this gap, it is suggested that the clinician and the client engage in an acting out of the scenes in the hierarchies. This type of activity is a form of psychodrama, except, of course, that the improvisations are centered around the scenes from the hierarchies. The clinician should rely on the reciprocal inhibitor for control. The goal is to eliminate negative emotion as a client response in stimulus situations.

Real-Life Situations

When control of difficult scenes has been clearly established, the clinician and client should discuss the experiments to be undertaken away from the clinic. In principle, the structure should not vary from the clinic scenes, but it will because of the ever-changing nature of life situations. The experiences of the client should be reported back in detail to the clinician and analyzed. Many of the new experiences can be incorporated into new hierarchies, which can then be presented in the clinic and rehearsed in improvisation.

By carefully carrying out this type of program, vocal behavior can eventually be modified through eradicating much of the tension produced by negative emotion.

SUMMARY

The three special procedures presented in this chapter by no means cover all of the "wholistic" approaches to voice training. Many voice specialists prefer to use a complete, sequential program of voice and diction reeducation, commencing with relaxation and breathing and including such topical areas as voice production, resonation, prosody, and integrating vocal skills. Other specialists are known to concentrate upon a given aspect of voice training, for example, the breath-sigh approach, or the proprioceptive-tactile-kinesthetic approach, exclusively, and use the procedure as the chief means of modifying vocal behavior.

The authors have strongly recommended that clinicians utilize assessment and training procedures that are specific to the problem, as presented in Chapters 2–5. Whatever approach is used, the clinician is urged to pursue his training program with the thoroughness and faithfulness the model deserves.

Index

Hyponasality, 12, 60–62, 183–184
Hypovalved larynx, 8
Hysterical aphonia, 40–41

Immature voice, 42, 53
Inharmonic, 7
Initial contact, nature of, 15
Instruction, 27
Intensity, 45

Jacobson, E., 114
Juvenile voice, 42, 53

Kennedy, J. F., 100
Kingsley, C., 108–109
Kipling, R., 143, 165

Labeling, description of, 3
Laryngeal
    amplitude, 45
    events, clusters of, 48
    noise, 10, 45–46
    oscillation, 9
    turbulence, 6
    valving, 7, 18, 35–36
        sporadic changes in, 7–8, 35–41
Laryngectomee, 47
Larynx
    amplitude, 45
    contributions of, 35
    frequency generation, 42
    noise generation, 45
    valving, 8, 18, 35
Lincoln, A., 165
Longfellow, H. W., 144, 197
Loudness, 38, 45

Metallic, 39
Mixta, 12, 61–62
Modal frequency (pitch), 71
Modifying target behaviors, 28
Modulation, 5

Mother Goose, 196
Muffled speech, 54
Mushy, 54

Nasal air turbulence, 13, 59
Nasal coupling, 11–13, 54
    negative, 60–62
    positive
        constant hypernasality II, 57–59
        constant hypernasality III, 59–60
        partial hypernasality I, 56–57
Nasality, definition of, 54–55
Nasal
    passage
        coupling, 11–13, 54
        emission, 13, 59
        resonators, 11–12
        uncoupling, 11–13
    resonance, 11–12
    speech, 58
Noise, laryngeal, 10, 45–46

Optimal cavity coupling, 56
Optimally valved larynx, 8
Optimum pitch, 65–71
Oscillation
    inappropriate shifts in, 43
    laryngeal, 9
    mode of, 9–10, 42

Paracode
    definition of, 1
    disorders, description of, 2–3
    variables, 2
Pharyngo-nasal, 51
Pharyngo-oral, 49–50
Phonation
    adducted (sporadic), 40–41
    characteristics of, 7
    hypervalvular, 39
    hypovalvular, 37
    initiating, 148
Phonetic power, 184
Physiology, 3

74 75 76 77 9 8 7 6 5 4 3 2 1